Helping Your Overweight Child:

A Do-It-Yourself Guide

Myung K. Park, MD, FAAP, FACC

Professor Emeritus (Pediatric Cardiology)

Former Chief of Pediatric Cardiology

Former Director of Preventive Cardiology and
Weight Management Clinic,

University of Texas Health Science Center,

San Antonio, Texas

ISBN: 1502328933

ISBN 13: 9781502328939

Library of Congress Control Number: 2014916272

LCCN Imprint Name: **City and State (If applicable)**

Dedication

Dedicated to my loving wife, Issun

CONTENTS

Acknowledgements

I thank my son, Christophe Y. Park, MD, PhD, who has given me a number of constructive suggestions, both for the contents of the book and in editing the manuscript.

I would like to thank Maribel Castro, my former assistant, and Linda Lopez, clinic manager at the Driscoll Specialty Clinic in McAllen, Texas, for encouraging me to write this book for concerned parents with overweight children. MS. Castro read an earlier version of the manuscript and provided me with constructive suggestions.

I would like to thank my former patients and their parents in my clinics in San Antonio and McAllen, Texas, for providing moments of joy of success and for sharing their experiences and inspiration along the long journey they took for healthy weight and better health for the family.

Preface

The epidemic of obesity in the United States and around the world, especially among children and adolescents, is one of the most pressing public health issues. Obesity contributes to the development of heart disease, diabetes, and many other chronic diseases. Even though nearly half of all American children and adolescents are either overweight or obese, little medical help is available to them and their families. Government and private efforts to prevent obesity are limited and largely ineffective. New efforts include First Lady Michelle Obama's "Let's Move" campaign, the new food guide system, the new school lunch program, and other government programs intended to increase children's opportunities for physical activity and improve their access to high-quality foods. These multifaceted approaches have the potential to alter the course of childhood obesity, but such programs take time to achieve noticeable success. More importantly, they do not focus on the most critical components of the epidemic: the child and his or her family.

Many concerned parents want to help improve the health of their obese children. They know that lifestyle changes, such as eating healthy foods and exercising regularly, are the keys to preventing and managing obesity. However, many do not have the knowledge to help their children establish a healthy lifestyle. Although healthcare professionals can play an important part in this process, the medical community is unfortunately not well prepared to address the epidemic. Most physicians do not provide services in the area of obesity prevention and management, and for various reasons, many communities do not have weight-management personnel or facilities. Few books have been written on childhood obesity, and even fewer books with concise, easy-to-use guides have been written specifically for parents. Concerned parents of overweight children have few places to turn for help. This book is intended to fill that void.

Parents of overweight children can do something to help their children. Recent research by Dr. Moria Golan and her coworkers in Israel and Dr. Anthea Magarey and her coworkers in Australia offer encouragement for parents of obese children. These studies show that trained parents can effectively manage the weight problems of their preadolescent children (Golan et al. 1998; Margarey et al. 2011). As long as parents are educated and motivated, the results can be as good as or better than those of weight-management clinics. The parents' know-how, guidance, and motivation will lead their children to success. This book was written to enhance these critical components of the parents' toolbox. Additional benefits of parental involvement include progress on the parents' weight, cholesterol, and blood pressure. The health of the whole family will improve.

Parents' motivation is essential. You, the parent, must be committed to helping your obese child. Children are not born knowing how to eat healthy or exercise regularly. If your child is obese, it is because he or she does not possess the information and resources necessary to develop a healthy lifestyle. By reading this book, you arm yourself with the knowledge to make this change.

This book is based on my experience as the director of the Preventive Cardiology and Weight Management Clinics for Children at the University of Texas Health Science Center in San Antonio. By working with families, I have seen firsthand how partnering with a knowledgeable healthcare provider can dramatically improve outcomes in childhood weight management. Unfortunately, it became apparent to me that many families did not have the knowledge to improve their lifestyles. To address this problem, I decided to "bring the clinic into the home" and empower parents as healthcare providers for their children.

In the following pages, I will describe in detail what a skilled medical professional would do for you and your overweight child in a specialized weight-management clinic. This book provides you with the information you need to guide your child through his or her day-to-day weight-control efforts and to counsel your child when he or she encounters difficulties. This book is like having an experienced healthcare provider in your home. The success you and your child will experience depends on your know-how and ability to guide your child to healthier eating and exercise habits.

The first part of the book describes what you need to know about childhood obesity, and provides a "do-it-yourself" guide to follow. The second part contains more advanced concepts and information that may help your child make healthy lifestyle choices.

Congratulations on deciding to do something about your child's weight problem. I wish you every success in improving your child's health!

Myung K. Park, MD, FAAP, FACC
San Antonio, Texas

Part 1

Basics of Home-Based Weight Management in Children

In part 1, the basic techniques of home-based weight-control efforts are presented for parents who plan to help their overweight child. The methods presented are the same as those used by most weight-management clinics for children. Weight clinics vary in approach, but they are all consistent with the recommendations of the Expert Committee on Childhood Obesity convened by the American Medical Association (AMA), the Department of Health and Human Services (HHS) Health Resources and Services Administration (HRSA), and the Centers for Disease Control and Prevention (CDC).

I will describe the steps that my staff and I take and the counseling we would offer if you brought your child to my clinic for help. By reading this part, you will learn how to help your overweight child and may yourself become an expert in managing children with weight problems.

Chapter 1

Overview of Childhood Obesity

If you want to help your overweight child, especially without the direct supervision of professionals, you need to know some basic facts about obesity. This chapter will help you to better understand the concepts and strategies that appear in later chapters.

What Does It Mean to Be Overweight or Obese?

A person is considered overweight or obese when he or she has excess body fat. While the terms *overweight* and *obese* have similar meanings, they differ in degree; overweight people are not as overweight as obese people.

Obese > Overweight

To determine whether a person is overweight or obese, most doctors use a measure known as body mass index (BMI). The BMI is a measure of body weight that takes height into account, which is a relevant factor because taller people tend to weigh more than shorter people. The BMI is used to categorize weight status as overweight or obese. The method used for calculating BMI is presented in chapter 2.

How Prevalent is Obesity?

Obesity is one of the most pressing public health issues today in the United States. Between 1980 and 2002, the prevalence of adult obesity doubled. The frequency of obesity in children and adolescents tripled in the same time period. According to statistics from the National Health and Nutrition Examination Survey, conducted in 2011–2012, 16.9 percent of children and adolescents (two to nineteen years old) and 34.9 percent of adults in the United States are obese. In addition, approximately 32 percent of children and adolescents are overweight. Therefore, nearly half of all American children and adolescents are either overweight or obese (Ogden et al. 2014, 806–816).

What Causes Children to Become Overweight?

Although genetic factors play a role in obesity, an unhealthy lifestyle has a greater influence. The two most important causes are excess caloric intake and not enough physical activity to use (or "burn") the calories taken in. The combination of excess caloric intake and inadequate physical activity causes a person to become overweight or obese.

Large Calorie versus Small Calorie as Units of Energy

"Calorie" is a unit of heat used to indicate the amount of energy that foods will produce in the human body. The term is used for two units of energy. The small calorie (symbol: cal) is the approximate amount of energy needed to raise the temperature of 1 gram of water by 1 degree Celsius. The small calorie unit is too small to describe calories in food. The large Calorie—also known as food calorie, dietary calorie, nutritional calorie, kilocalorie, or Calorie, capital C (symbol: Cal)—is the amount of energy needed to raise the temperature of 1 kg of water by 1 degree Celsius. One food calorie or large calorie (Calorie) is equal to 1,000 small calories or 1 kilocalorie (symbol: kcal) (i.e., 1 Calorie = 1 kcal = 1,000 calories).

Energy Balance

You need to understand the concept of energy balance; this is very basic in understanding obesity. Your body weight is determined by the number of calories (or units of energy) you take in from food and the number of calories you burn from physical activity each day. When you eat, you take in calories, and every time you engage in a physical activity, you use calories.

- When you eat the same number of calories as your body uses, your weight stays the same (A in fig. 1.1).

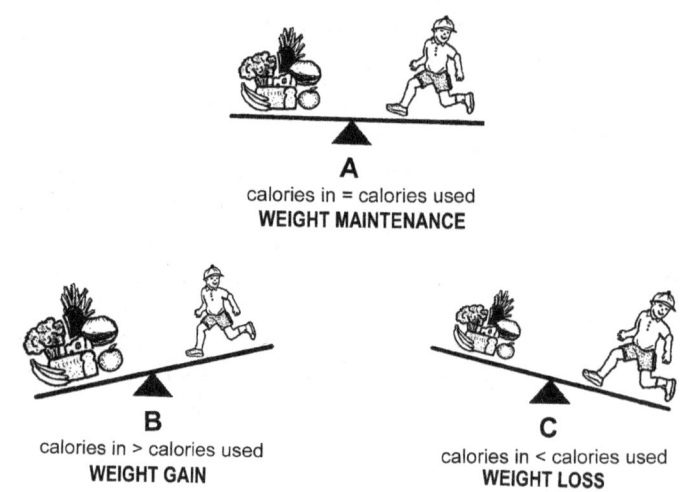

A
calories in = calories used
WEIGHT MAINTENANCE

B
calories in > calories used
WEIGHT GAIN

C
calories in < calories used
WEIGHT LOSS

Figure 1.1. Energy balance (> means "greater than," < means "less than," and = means "equals").

- When you eat more calories than you burn, you have a *positive energy balance*. Your body will store the extra calories in the form of fat, and you will gain weight (B in fig. 1.1). When you have a positive energy balance on a regular basis, you will become overweight or obese.
- When you eat fewer calories than you use, you have a *negative energy balance*. Your body uses stored calories faster than you replenish them, and you may lose weight (C in fig. 1.1).

An overweight or obese child has repeatedly consumed more calories than his or her body can use. Even though you may think your child is not consuming excess calories, one thing is clear: your overweight child has taken in more calories than he or she could burn for some period of time. He or she must have unhealthy eating habits, has not had enough exercise to burn the calories, or both.

What Are Unhealthy Eating Habits?

Unhealthy eating habits include consuming too many unhealthy foods with large number of calories and too few healthy foods.

- Unhealthy foods include solid fats, added sugars, and sodium (SoFAS).
- Healthy foods include fruits, vegetables, high-fiber whole grains, low-fat milk and dairy products, and seafood.

SoFAS is an acronym used by the US government in its 2010 dietary guidelines. It stands for solid fat and added sugars (and salts). Health experts recommend that SoFAS should account for no more than 5–15 percent of your daily calories. Americans of all ages and genders get closer to 35 percent of their daily calories from SoFAS. Heavy doses of SoFAS come from eating at restaurants, especially fast-food outlets.

Fats that are solid at room temperature include saturated and trans fats. Trans fat, also known as trans fatty acids, is an unhealthy solid fat, made through the chemical process of hydrogenation of liquid oils. Saturated fats are found primarily in animal products (meat, butter, cheese, and milk) and rarely in plants (coconut and palm oil). Trans fats are often found in prepackaged snacks, baked goods, and fried foods (chips, cookies, donuts, and cakes). Examples of solid fats include butter, milk fat, beef fat (tallow and suet), chicken fat, cream, pork fat (lard), stick margarine, shortening, hydrogenated and partially hydrogenated oils, and coconut and palm oils. Examples of products with added sugar include soda, energy drinks, cookies, cake, fruit drinks, ice cream, candy, and cinnamon rolls. Too much salt intake also contributes to weight gain.

Among all three macronutrients (defined as foodstuffs that provide energy or calories), fat and oil supply more calories than protein and carbohydrates. One gram of fat (or oil) gives you nine Calories of energy, while the same amount of carbohydrate and protein gives you four Calories. This is why intake of high-fat food should be reduced in weight-control efforts.

How Important Is Physical Activity?

Physical activity is an integral component of energy balance. Physical activity burns calories and thus helps prevent weight problems. A sedentary lifestyle may cause weight gain because fewer calories are burned. All weight-management programs emphasize increasing physical activity. Any form of physical activity, whether a planned exercise or simply playing outdoors, burns calories. For children, lack of physical activity is often the result of spending too much time watching television, playing computer games, or working on a computer.

What Are the Consequences of Being Obese?

The major diseases associated with adult obesity are hypertension, heart disease, diabetes, and certain types of cancer. Less well-known complications include stroke, liver disorders, gallbladder disease, pulmonary function impairment, endocrine abnormalities, pregnancy complications, trauma to the weight-bearing joints, gout, skin disease, and proteinuria (protein in the urine).

Even though some obese children may appear healthy and do not have diabetes or heart disease, it is likely that these conditions are in their early stages in their bodies. Obese children and adolescents frequently exhibit high levels of cholesterol and triglycerides, high blood pressure, and low levels of HDL ("good") cholesterol, all of which increase their risk of heart disease in adulthood. Obese children exhibit early signs of diabetes, including high levels of blood insulin and a skin condition called acanthosis nigricans (fig. 1.2). They are more likely to have asthma and sleep disorders. Some complications are common, while others are rare but serious. All of these complications can significantly worsen your overweight child's health, and it is better to prevent them from occurring. Even children and adolescents who are merely overweight, but not obese, are at risk of developing health problems.

Selected complications of obesity seen in children and adolescents are listed below. Most of them can be diagnosed only through a physical exam and laboratory tests.

- One out of three obese children has high blood pressure (hypertension). The majority of children with high blood pressure are also obese.
- High levels of cholesterol and/or triglyceride and low levels of HDL cholesterol are common. They all increase the risk of heart disease. When these conditions occur in association with borderline elevation of blood glucose, the condition is called "metabolic syndrome." Metabolic syndrome often develops into type 2 diabetes and heart disease. This syndrome may be seen in more than 30 percent of obese children and in more than 50 percent of severely obese adolescents.
- High levels of plasma insulin (known as hyperinsulinemia) are found in about 25 percent of obese children. This condition usually precedes type 2 diabetes.
- Acanthosis nigricans is frequently seen in obese children and adolescents. It is characterized by a patch of skin with dark streaks that cannot be washed off. The condition is commonly seen in the neck (fig. 1.2) but sometimes also in the armpits

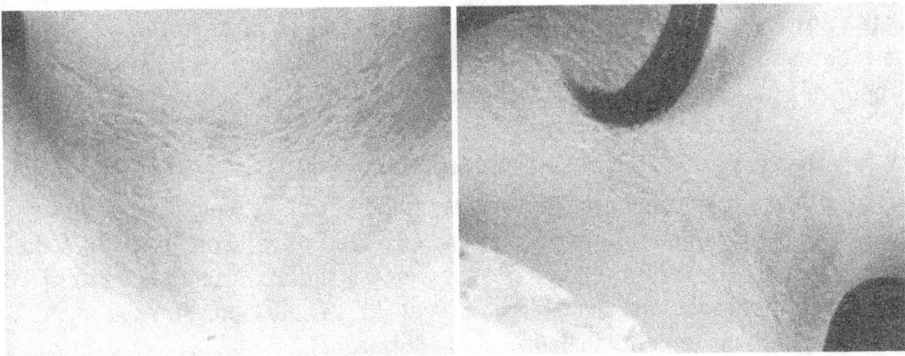

Figure 1.2. Acanthosis nigricans of the neck in a fifteen-year-old girl. Left: front view. Right: side view. (Source: US Public Health Services, "Acanthosis nigricans." www.dphhs.mt.gov/publichealth/diabetes/documents/AcanBrochure.pdf.)

and abdominal area. It is a risk factor for developing diabetes, and nearly 90 percent of children with type 2 diabetes have the condition.

- Obese children and adolescents experience asthma attacks more often than in nonobese children and have more difficulty controlling their asthma symptoms.

- Evidence of liver damage is seen in some obese children, which is due to accumulation of fat in the liver. This condition is known as nonalcoholic fatty liver disease (NAFLD) or hepatic steatosis. As many as 25–50 percent of obese children may have evidence of the disease, according to some reports (Manco et al. 2008, 667–676). Obese children often develop type 2 diabetes. Normal-weight individuals rarely develop type 2 diabetes. The frequency of children developing type 2 diabetes increases in parallel with the increase in the prevalence of obesity.

- Sleep disorders, such as obstructive sleep apnea (blockage of airway passages with difficulty sleeping soundly at night), appear in about 5 percent of children with severe obesity. Common signs of the disorder include loud snoring (with periods of silence followed by gasps), restless sleep, and excessive daytime sleepiness.

- Orthopedic problems are more common in obese children. Knee and ankle injuries occur more frequently in obese children than nonobese children. Some obese children have bowing of the leg bones (Blount disease), joint damage (slipped capital femoral epiphyses), or back problems.

- Polycystic ovary syndrome may be seen in obese adolescent girls who have absent or irregular menses (fewer than nine cycles per year). They may present with increased hair growth, excessive acne, and acanthosis nigricans. These patients often develop type 2 diabetes.

- Pseudotumor cerebri is an extremely rare but serious condition that occurs more commonly in obese children, and it is due to increased pressure in the skull. The most common symptom is headaches, often associated with vomiting, blurred or double vision, and an increased sensitivity to light. When this condition is suspected, it requires an urgent diagnostic work-up and treatment.

- At the psychological level, overweight or obese children often have low self-esteem, exhibit eating disorders (particularly in white girls), are the victims of bullying, and report feelings of depression, estrangement, and embarrassment.

How Are Overweight and Obese Children Managed?

Although obese adults often put themselves on a diet to lose weight, no diets are used in the weight management of obese children. Such diets never work in children. Sudden, drastic reductions in caloric intake do not work in adults in the long term either. Currently, no medicines are available or proven to be safe and effective in the initial stage of weight management in children and adolescents.

The best—and probably the only—way for your child to reduce his or her weight is by making lifestyle changes. Most successful pediatric weight-management programs employ strategies to achieve a healthy lifestyle.

What Is a Healthy Lifestyle?

The bottom line for weight management for both adults and children is to "eat healthy and exercise." Most people have heard this message, but many people have difficulty grasping its full meaning. To help people better understand what constitutes healthy habits, some simple guidelines have been developed. One of these is the "5-2-1-0" message developed by the New Hampshire Health Department (fig. 1.3). It is easy to understand and remember:

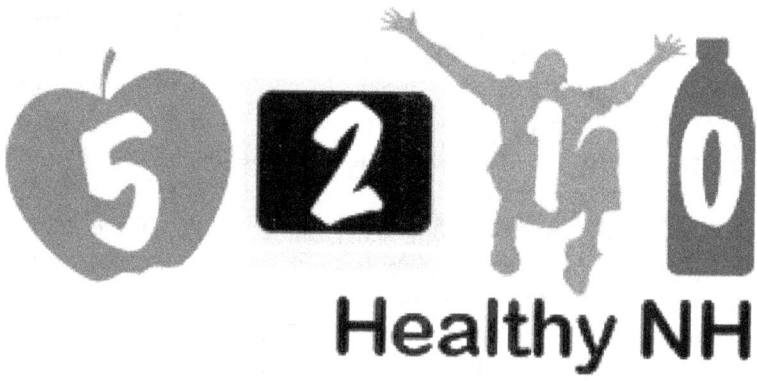

Figure 1.3. The 5-2-1-0 Message. (Source: Foundation for Healthy Communities, "the 5-2-1-0 NH." Reproduced by permission from the Foundation for Healthy Communities, http://www.healthynh.com.)

- **5**—Eat at least five servings of fruits and vegetables most days.
- **2**—Limit "screen time" to two hours or less daily. Screen time refers to time spent in front of a screen—including watching television, playing video games, and using the computer.
- **1**—Participate in one or more hours of physical activity every day.
- **0**—Avoid soda and sugar-sweetened drinks. Instead, drink water and low-fat or fat-free milk.

What Is Healthy Eating?

People are confused about what "healthy eating" is and cannot clearly visualize it. In June 2011, the US Department of Agriculture (USDA) introduced a food guide system called MyPlate (fig. 1.4) that makes it easy for consumers to understand what a healthy plate should look like. Recall the adage "a picture is worth a thousand words." It is important to familiarize yourself with this icon because it will help you tremendously in your effort to provide your child with a healthy diet.

MyPlate divides a plate into four sections that show what a balanced meal should look like.

- Fruits and vegetables take up half the plate.
- A quadrant on the other side is assigned for grains.
- The last quadrant is assigned for protein.
- Dairy is seen to the side in a blue circle (much like a cup).

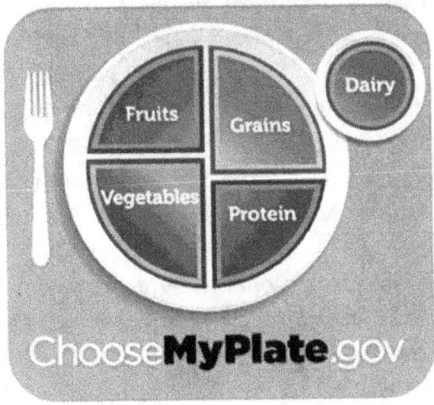

Figure 1.4. MyPlate, the new food guide system.
(Source: US Department of Agriculture, "USDA's MyPlate,"
http://www.choosemyplate.gov/images/MyPlateImages/JPG/myplate_green.jpg.)

The dominant message of MyPlate concerns plant-based foods. Fruits, vegetables, and grains cover three-quarters of the plate. The remaining quadrant is assigned to protein. Note that protein does not have to be of animal origin like beef, pork, chicken, or fish. Protein of plant origin, such as beans, peas, and tofu, is equally good. For most Americans, however, it is unrealistic to eat half a plate of fruits and vegetables every day. Still, the idea is to eat as closely to the MyPlate icon as possible, which will result in reduced consumption of SoFAS.

What Are the Targets of Weight-Control Efforts?

In summarizing what we have discussed so far, common targets of lifestyle changes used in weight-management efforts for children include the following:

1. Increasing consumption of fruits, vegetables, and whole-grain food products
2. Decreasing physical inactivity by limiting TV, computer, and video game time (less than two hours a day)
3. Increasing physical activities to more than sixty minutes daily
4. Limiting consumption of high-sugar foods and beverages such as cakes and soda
5. Limiting consumption of high-fat foods such as fast food, fried food, and chips
6. Limiting frequency of eating at restaurants, especially fast-food restaurants

These are easy to remember, because the first four are the components of the 5-2-1-0 message. The fifth and sixth entries aim to limit consumption of SoFAS. These behavioral changes will result in reduced caloric intake and increased calorie burning, resulting in reduction of weight (i.e., negative energy balance).

What Are the Ingredients of Successful Weight Management?

Lifestyle changes are the best way to control weight problems, but they do not come easily. They are more likely to succeed when they include the following components:

- Knowledge. Parents and the overweight child should know about obesity and weight-management strategies.
- Commitment and support of parents and family. Without the support of parents and family, the effort is less likely to succeed, even within in a professional weight-clinic setting.
- Professional supervision. In professional weight-management clinics, physicians and/or trained healthcare providers supervise overweight children and their parents. In parent-initiated weight-management efforts, books like this one will provide you with the knowledge to help your child successfully control weight problems. However, it is strongly advised that you inform your child's doctor of your planned action and ask for her support.

How Will This Book Help You?

The methods in this book are similar to those used by professional weight-management clinics, with the exception of physical exams and laboratory tests. With the knowledge gained by reading this book and carefully following the plans provided, your success may be as good as or better than taking your child to a weight-loss clinic.

It is critically important to prepare yourself mentally to tackle your child's weight problem. Without your commitment, the problem cannot be solved. Even if you take your child to a weight-management clinic, you still have to do your part. The professionals will ask you to take more or less the same actions as those outlined in this book.

The remaining chapters of part 1 provide a "do-it-yourself guide" that is the same as those provided by weight clinics. It achieves the following:

- Determines the severity of your child's weight status. Is he or she overweight or obese?
- Assesses your child's risk factors for diabetes and coronary heart disease. This will give you an idea of the degree of urgency required for action.
- Identifies the lifestyle that may have contributed to your child's weight problem. This will be done by asking you thirty questions about your child and family's lifestyle.
- Provides advice on each topic in your child and family's lifestyle questionnaires. This chapter describes why some of your child's behaviors are unhealthy and how you can correct them. This chapter is like a "live-in counselor."
- Describes day-to-day and step-by-step management schemes with ample examples, including the following:

  1) Setting goals to correct unhealthy lifestyles
  2) Monitoring the progress your child is making on a regular basis
  3) Tackling problems you may run into, including setbacks and obesity-related complications

Part 2 covers these important topics:

- Chapter 10 provides advanced knowledge about a number of obesity-related topics. It is not necessary to read the chapter at the beginning of your weight-control efforts, but its insights will enhance your understanding of a number of obesity-related questions.
- Chapter 11 describes medications and surgeries that are available only at approved weight-management clinics.

The appendices include tables, figures, and forms, available for quick reference during weight-management efforts.

Chapter 2

Weight Status and Risk Factors

Let's begin by checking whether your child is overweight or obese. We will then determine if other members of your family have weight problems, as well as learn about your child's risk of developing heart disease or diabetes.

Know Your Child's Weight Status

The simplest way of knowing whether a person is overweight or obese is to calculate body mass index (BMI). BMI takes height into account. Although it can overestimate fat mass in trained athletes or muscular individuals, BMI is accepted internationally as the screening method of choice for identifying people who are overweight or obese.

How to Calculate BMI

The formulas to calculate BMI differ depending on the units used to measure height and weight. One uses meters (m) and kilograms (kg), and the other uses inches (in.) and pounds (lb.). There are also convenient tables available to approximate BMI values.

- Method 1: BMI = weight in kilograms / (height in meters x height in meters)
- Method 2: BMI = weight in pounds / (height in inches x height in inches) x 703
- Method 3: Tables A.1(a) and A.1(b) in the appendix

How to Categorize the Degree of Excess Weight

Once you have calculated the BMI, it is simple to determine whether a person is overweight or obese (see table 2.1).

- For an adult, a BMI of 30 or more is obese; a BMI between 25 and 29.9 is overweight. A BMI of 40 or more is severe obesity.
- Because children keep growing in height and increasing in weight, single sets of numbers cannot be used for them. The BMI values need to be checked against established BMI percentile curves that vary depending on age and gender (see figs. A.1 and A.2). A BMI between the 85th and 95th percentile for age and gender

- qualifies for the *overweight* category, and those greater than the 95th percentile qualify for the *obesity* category. A BMI in the 99th percentile or greater is

Table 2.1 Classification of weight status by BMI in adults and children

BODY COMPOSITION	ADULTS	CHILDREN & ADOLESCENTS
Underweight	Less than 18.5	Less than the 5th percentile
Normal weight	18.5–24.9	Between the 5th and 85th percentiles
Overweight	25.0–29.9	Between the 85th and 95th percentile
Obese	Greater than 30.0	Higher than the 95th percentile
Severely obese	Greater than 40.0	The 99th percentile and higher

considered in the *severe obesity* range (see table 2.1). Table A.2 provides the 85th, 95th, and 99th percentile values for boys and girls according to age. You can use this table to categorize a child's weight status instead of plotting the BMI value on a graph as shown in fig. 2.1.

Example of BMI Calculation and Categorization

George is an eleven-year-old boy who weighs 59.1 kg (130 lb.) and is 1.4 m (55 in.) tall.

1. Determine George's BMI using the different methods presented above.

   - Method 1: BMI = 59.1 ÷ (1.4 x 1.4) = 59.1 / 1.96 = 30.15
   - Method 2: BMI = 130 / (55 x 55) x 703 = 130 / 3,025 x 703 = 0.042975 x 703 = 30.2
   - Method 3: Refer to tables A.1(a) and A.1(b). You will find an appropriate height in inches in the left-hand column. Move across to find a weight closest to your weight, and the BMI is at the top of the column. The National Heart, Lung, and Blood Institute's table starts at 58 in. Therefore, this method cannot be used for George.

2. Categorize George's weight status

George's BMI is 30.2. When his BMI is plotted on fig. A.1, it is way above the 95th percentile and in the severe obesity range (fig. 2.1). His BMI is much greater than the 97th percentile, the top curve. He is close to the 99th percentile (see table A.2 for the 99th percentile value). According to table A.2, the 99th percentile value for an eleven-year-old boy is 30.7. Therefore, George is nearly severely obese.

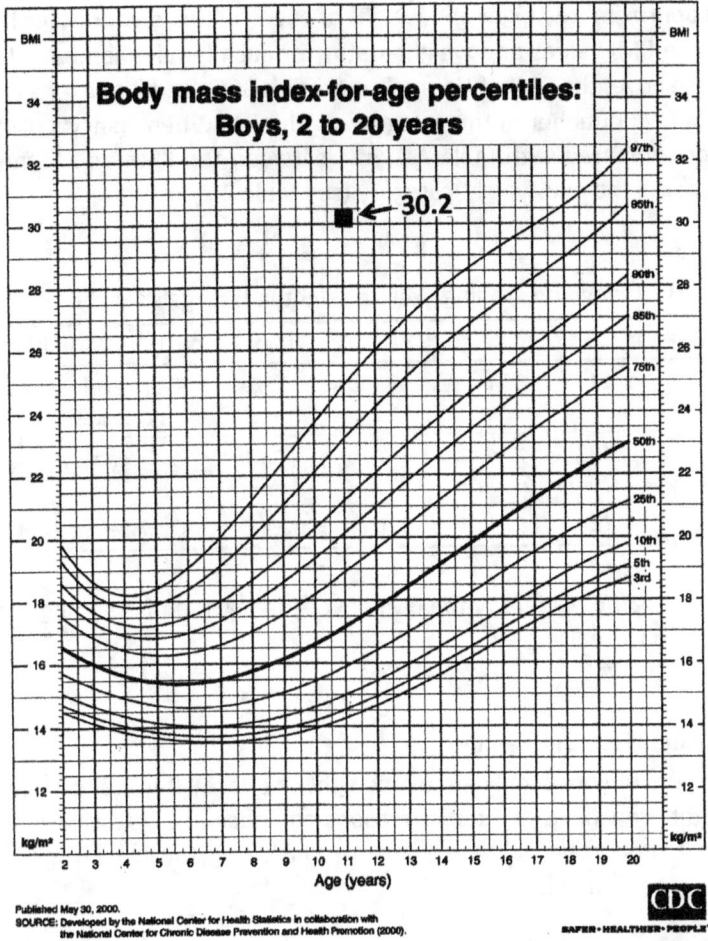

Figure 2.1. George's BMI of 30.2 is plotted. He is near severely obese. (Source: The National Center for Health Statistics, in collaboration with the National Center for Chronic Disease Prevention and Health Promotion, "Body Mass Index-for-Age," 2000.)

Obesity in the Family

This may be a good time to find out who in your family is overweight or obese. Frequently, more than one person in a family has a weight problem, because family members share genes and are exposed to similar living environments. When more than one member of the family is obese, the situation may call for recruiting other overweight family members and using a more aggressive approach.

Finding BMI and Weight Status in George's Family

An example of finding out family members' BMI is presented in table 2.2 for George's family, which includes his mother and his sister, Nancy.

- Record the approximate height and weight of each person in your household.
- Determine the BMI values and weight status for each family member. Using one of the methods above, the BMI of George's mother is 30.2, and his sister's is 23.8.
- His mother's BMI puts her in the category of obesity. When Nancy's BMI is plotted in fig. A.2 or compared with table A.2, it is between the 85th and 95th percentile, which puts her in the overweight category (see table 2.2).

Table 2.2 Calculating and grading excess weight in George's family

RELATIONSHIP	AGE	HEIGHT	WEIGHT	BMI	WEIGHT STATUS
George	11	55 in.	130 lb.	30.2	Near severely Obese
Mother	42	5 ft. 4 in. (64 in.)	176 lb.	30.2	Obese
Sister (Nancy)	12	57 in.	110 lb.	23.8	Overweight

After studying this example, identify the BMI of your family members using the method that you have found the easiest.

What Are the Results for Your Family?

How many members of your family are overweight or obese? If more than one member has excess weight, you have additional reasons to proceed aggressively with weight management. It is important to have everyone, including those who are not obese, participate and support the efforts.

Some medical conditions, such as hypothyroidism, can cause obesity in children. Make sure that each overweight/obese member of your family is evaluated by a physician.

Some medications can contribute to weight gain. If your child has been on a medication on a long-term basis, check with your doctor for its potential contribution to your child's weight problem. Examples of such medications include high-dose corticosteroids, allergy medicines (Periactin), seizure medicines (valproate), antidepressants (imipramine, amitriptyline, trazodone), and antipsychotic drugs (Zyprexa, Risperdal, Seroquel, Geodon).

Some genetic conditions can be associated with obesity (see table A.3 for their clinical features). Note that most of the genetic conditions are associated with developmental disabilities and small stature.

Assessment of Risk Factors

Being overweight or obese is a significant risk factor for diabetes and heart disease (there are other risk factors for these conditions as well). The more risk factors you have, the more likely your chance of developing a disease. It is a good idea to check your child's (and other family members') risk factors for heart disease and diabetes at this time.

Your child's doctor needs to be involved at this stage. To assess your child's risk factors for developing heart disease or diabetes, have your child's doctor order tests, such as those for blood glucose and a lipid profile that includes low-density lipoprotein or LDL cholesterol, high-density lipoprotein or HDL cholesterol, and triglycerides. Measure your child's blood pressure, and check for signs of risk factors such as acanthosis nigricans.

Risk Factors for Heart Disease

Heart disease is not a major cause of death among children and adolescents, but it is the largest cause of death among adults in the United States. It is well established that the onset of atherosclerotic heart disease occurs in late childhood and adolescence, and preventive efforts should start at that time. Known risk factors for heart disease are listed in box 2.1. Note that obesity is one of the risk factors for heart disease. Your child's doctor needs to check whether your child has high blood pressure or abnormal blood cholesterol levels.

Box 2.1   Risk factors for heart disease

- Family history of premature heart disease, stroke, or peripheral vascular disease (before age 55 years in men and before 65 years in women).
  Include parents, uncles and aunts, and grandparents on both sides of the family.
- High blood pressure (hypertension)*
- High cholesterol (hypercholesterolemia)*
- Low levels of high-density lipoprotein (HDL) cholesterol*
- Smoking
- Obesity

Presence of three or more risk factors constitutes risk of developing heart disease.

* Your doctor needs to check if your child has these conditions.
Sources: "Summary of the third report of the national cholesterol education program (NCEP) expert panel on detection, education, and treatment of high blood cholesterol in adults (adult treatment panel III) final report." *Circulation* 106 (2002): 3143–3421.

Does your child have two or more of these risk factors? If so, your child is at risk of developing heart disease.

Some risk factors, like family history of heart disease, are not modifiable, but other factors, such as obesity, high blood pressure, and high cholesterol levels, are modifiable or treatable. Weight-control efforts should start now.

If your teenage child or any adult family member is a smoker, he or she should stop smoking. Smoking is one of the more important risk factors for heart disease. You may need advice from a physician or a smoking-cessation professional on how to quit.

Diabetes Risk Factors

Risk factors for developing type 2 diabetes are shown in box 2.2. In this case, there are more risk factors than those for heart disease. Obese female adolescents of ethnic minorities are at particularly high risk of developing type 2 diabetes. Your child's doctor needs to check him or her for acanthosis nigricans and blood pressure levels and order laboratory tests for blood sugar, cholesterols, and triglyceride levels.

Box 2.2 Risk factors for type 2 diabetes

- Obesity
- Family history of type 2 diabetes (include child's parents, uncles and aunts, and grandparents on both sides of the family)
- Ethnic minority (e.g., African American, Mexican American, American Indian, Asian or Pacific Islander descent)
- Puberty (The mean age at the time of diagnosis is 13.5 years)
- Female gender
- Features of the metabolic syndrome
  - High blood pressure*
  - HDL-cholesterol, 40 mg/dL or lower*
  - Fasting glucose, 100 mg/dL or greater*
  - Triglyceride 150 mg/dL or greater*
- Acanthosis nigricans

If your child is overweight or obese and you answered "yes" to two or more of the remaining risk factors, your child is at risk of developing type 2 diabetes.

---

* Your doctor needs to confirm these diagnoses.

Modified from S. Arslanian, "Type 2 diabetes in children: clinical aspects and risk factors." *Hormone Research* 57, Suppl. 1 (2002): 19–28.

Does your child have two or more of the remaining four risk factors? If so, intervention is urgent.

Risk factors such as family history of diabetes, ethnicity, age, and gender cannot be changed. Managing weight is the only feasible way to reduce the risk of developing diabetes. Weight control can also increase HDL cholesterol and lower blood pressure levels, thereby reducing the risk of heart disease.

Metabolic Syndrome

In addition to the conventional risk factors for developing type 2 diabetes and heart disease, metabolic syndrome (also known as cardiometabolic syndrome or syndrome X) is a risk. It consists of clusters of risk factors that occur together (see box 2.3). It occurs more frequently in obese individuals, particularly those with abdominal obesity (excess fat around the waist and inside the abdomen), and many of them have hyperinsulinemia. Researchers have found that metabolic syndrome is present in 39 percent of moderately obese adolescents (BMI > 95th percentile) and in more than 50 percent of severely obese adolescents (BMI at the 99th percentile or more) (Singh 2006, 403-413) there are overlapping features between metabolic syndrome and the previously described risk factors for diabetes and heart disease.

The presence of metabolic syndrome signals a more serious risk of developing both diabetes and heart disease, because a person who has the syndrome is already in the prediabetic stage, in addition to having other risk factors for heart disease including high levels of triglycerides (hypertriglyceridemia). The prediabetic stage occurs before fully developed diabetes. At this stage, there is an impairment of carbohydrate metabolism similar to that seen in diabetes, but not all the diagnostic criteria for frank diabetes are satisfied. The presence of metabolic syndrome calls for more aggressive lifestyle changes than when only risk factors for diabetes or heart disease are present. Ask your child's doctor if your child has metabolic syndrome. Your child's doctor needs to check your child's blood pressure and order laboratory tests for triglycerides, HDL cholesterol, and glucose.

Unlike in adults, there were different proposed definitions of metabolic syndrome in children and adolescents. Box 2.3 lists the most recent definition, proposed by the International Diabetes Federation in 2007. This proposal was based on data from national health surveys that were unavailable when other, earlier proposals were made. In this proposal, the definition of the syndrome is the same as for adults.

Does your obese child meet the definition of metabolic syndrome? If so, it indicates that he or she has increased risks of developing diabetes and heart disease, which represents a more serious situation than the two other risk factor groups. Weight-control efforts should start now. Even if he or she does not have metabolic syndrome, you should not wait until things get worse. Review the results of the lab tests that your child's doctor has ordered.

Box 2.3 Proposed definition of the metabolic syndrome in children and adolescents

---

- Triglyceride, 150 mg/dL or greater
- HDL-cholesterol, 40 mg/dL or lower
- BMI, the 95th percentile and greater
  (or waist circumference greater than the 90th percentile*)
- Fasting glucose, 100 mg/dL or greater
- Systolic blood pressure, 90th percentile or greater*

The presence of at least three of the abnormalities constitute metabolic syndrome

---

*Your child's physician will have access to the 90th percentile values for waist circumference and systolic blood pressure.

Adapted from P. Zimmer P, G. Alberti, F. Kaufman et al, "The metabolic syndrome in children and adolescents." *Lancet* 369 (2007): 2059–2061.

A word of caution is due. Some parents of obese children may be happy to learn that their child's blood test results are normal. While they should be happy about those results, some parents take them to mean that their child is in the clear regarding obesity. This is a grave misunderstanding; it is only a matter of time before the child's cholesterol, blood sugar, and other measures will become abnormal. Their child is lucky that other damage has not taken place, but it is not going to stay that way. Obesity is bad enough, as it is the cornerstone of many chronic diseases. Regardless of the results of any laboratory tests, start weight-management efforts now.

By now, you should have a good idea of the severity of your child's excess weight, as well as your child's risk factors for developing diabetes and heart disease. Based on this information, you should understand the importance of weight control, as well as some of the consequences resulting from poor weight control during childhood. Because obesity is a risk factor for diabetes and heart disease and a component of metabolic syndrome, controlling weight is important. It cannot be stressed enough that the earlier healthy lifestyle habits begin, the better the health outcomes for your child and your family. When it comes to these diseases, prevention is always a better path to travel than treatment.

It is highly recommended that your child's doctor check your child's blood sugar, cholesterol, triglycerides, and blood pressure levels before starting weight-control efforts, and that the results remain handy for later comparison.

Chapter 3

Lifestyle Questionnaire

As mentioned earlier, lifestyle change is the cornerstone of weight management. To successfully change unhealthy habits, it is crucial that you find out which diet and activity practices have contributed to your child's weight problem. Table 3.1 includes thirty lifestyle questions for you to answer. For each question, circle the answer that best describes the lifestyle of your child and family. If you are making lifestyle assessments for multiple children, answer the questions separately for each child.

Table 3.1 Lifestyle questions

Physical Activity of Your Child		1	2	3	4
1	How many days a week (on average) does your child play outside for at least sixty minutes? Include time spent at school in physical education class, organized and unorganized activities, and house chores.	0–1	2–3	4–5	6–7
2	How many hours per day does your child watch TV/DVD/videotapes, work on computers, or play electronic games?	4 or more	3	2	0–1

Diet and Eating Behaviors of Your Child		1	2	3	4
3	How many days in a week does your child eat whole-grain cereals, oatmeal, or other whole grain products for breakfast and other meals?	0	1–2	3–5	More than 5
4	What kind of bread does your child eat at home?	White	Others	Whole-wheat (or other whole-grain)	
5	How many days in a week does your child eat potatoes (such as baked potatoes, mashed potato, or potato salad) as the main portion of a meal?	4 or more	2–3	1	0
6	How many days in a week does your child eat at least 1 ½ cups of fruits each day? (2 cups for adolescents)	0–1	2–3	4–5	6–7
7	How many days in a week does your child eat at least 2 ½ cups of vegetables each day (such as green, yellow, orange, or red vegetables)? (3 cups for adolescents) Do not include potatoes.	0–1	2–3	4–5	6–7
8	How many days in a week does your child eat vegetables (not potatoes) or sliced fruits as snacks?	0–1	2–3	4–5	6–7
9	What type of milk does your child drink?	Whole	2%	1%	Skim
10	How many days in a week does your child eat regular cheese (like American, cheddar, Swiss, Monterey jack) instead of low-fat or part skim cheeses as a snack or on sandwiches or pizza?	5–7	3–4	2	0–1
11	How many times a week does your child eat hamburgers or cheeseburgers? Include those eaten at the school cafeteria.	5 or more	3–4	2	0–1
12	How many times a week does your child eat French fries, hash browns, or tater tots? Include those eaten at the school cafeteria.	5 or more	3–4	2	0–1
13	How many times does your child eat fried food (such as fried chicken, fried fish, etc.) in a week?	4 or more	2–3	1	0

Table 3.1 Lifestyle questions (Continued.)

	Diet and Eating Behaviors of Your Child (Continued)	1	2	3	4
14	How many times per week does your child eat potato chips (and other kinds of chips)?	4 or more	3	2	0–1
15	How many times a day does your child eat sweets like cakes, pies, ice cream, cookies, pastries, donuts, muffins, chocolates, or candy?	4 or more	3	2	0–1
16	How many regular sodas (non diet) does your child consume each day?	3 or more	2	1	0
17	How many glasses of 100% fruit juice (such as orange juice) does your child drink in a day?	4 or more	3	2	0–1
18	How many glasses of fruit drinks or fruit juice cocktails (examples: Sunny Delight, Hi-C, Hawaiian Punch, lemonade, and many other fruit-flavored drinks) does your child drink in a day?	3 or more	2	1	0
19	How much would you say your child eats at each meal compared to their peers?	Very large	Large	Average	Small
20	How often does your child miss or skip breakfast?	Often	Sometimes	Rarely	Never
21	Does your child eat while watching TV?	Often	Sometimes	Rarely	Never
22	How often does your child eat bedtime snacks?	Often	Sometimes	Rarely	Never

	Family Knowledge and Lifestyle	1	2	3	4
23	How often do you read the nutrition facts (food labels) on food packages?	Never	Rarely	Sometimes	Often
24	When you buy meat, how often do you look for lean meats?	Rarely	Sometimes	Often	Always
25	How often do you deep fry or pan fry food when you cook?	Often	Sometimes	Rarely	Never
26	How often do you choose low-fat or fat-free varieties of food when you shop?	Rarely	Sometimes	Often	Always
27	How many times a week do you prepare a main dish that contains poultry or fish?	0–1	2	3	4 or more
28	How many times a week does your family eat at a sit-down restaurant or eat take-out food (prepared at a restaurant)?	4 or more	3	2	0–1
29	How many days in a week does the family eat a home-cooked dinner together?	1–2	3–4	5–6	7
30	How often do you have family outings on the weekends?	Never	Rarely	Sometimes	Often

What to Do with Your Answers

While you were answering the questions, you probably noticed that the answers are arranged in such a way that the most healthful (or best lifestyle behaviors) are in the rightmost columns. For each question, the answers in the two left cells represent behaviors that should be changed to appear like the actions reflected in the rightmost cells. Answers in the third column from the left are acceptable but may need improvement.

You also noticed that questions 1–22 deal with your child's lifestyle, while questions 23–30 reflect your family's lifestyle behaviors. Your child will have to make major efforts to change, so, likewise, change your family's lifestyle behaviors to the rightmost cells as quickly as you can. This will make your child's lifestyle changes easier; in fact, you may find they can be done without much pain to your child. He or she may not even notice certain changes.

Before you start, look at how your answers are distributed. This will give you some perspective on your current lifestyle and how urgent, difficult, or time consuming it will be to successfully change it.

- If the majority of your answers are in the two left columns, your child has many unhealthy behaviors to change. It may take more time and effort from everybody in the family to succeed.
- If the majority of your answers are in the two middle columns, it suggests that your child's behavior changes may be relatively easy and may take less time than the above situation.
- If the majority of your answers are in the two right columns, your child has relatively few unhealthy behaviors to change, but those few particular unhealthy habits may have caused the weight problem.

Chapter 4

Ready to Start

Before you embark on this journey, remember that changing unhealthy habits is a long journey for your child, you, and your family. Expect that there will be many starts, stops, and restarts, but if you are mentally and emotionally prepared to follow the plan described in this book and persevere for your child's sake, even when things are not going your way, you will be happy with the long-term results.

Before you begin, consider the following aspects of this lifestyle-change and weight-loss process:

- How urgent is it to control your child's weight problem?
- What approaches will be used in the weight-management efforts?
- What are the chances that your child will succeed in managing his weight?
- Are there advantages of a parent-guided weight-management effort such as the one you are trying?

Severity and Urgency

In general, the higher your child's BMI and the more the risk factors he or she has, the more urgent it is to initiate a weight-control program.

Does your child's BMI make him or her overweight or obese?

- If your child is overweight (BMI between the 85th and 95th percentile), it is important to take action to prevent him or her from becoming obese.
- If your child is obese (BMI in the 95th percentile or more), the time for action has come. Do not delay.
- If your child is at the high end of the obesity scale (BMI near or above the 99th percentile), the chances of successfully managing your child's weight are not as good as for less severely obese children. You may want to seek help at a supervised weight-control program. Regardless of whether you do this immediately, you can still start implementing some of the lifestyle changes you have learned from this book.
- Results of obesity treatment studies indicate that it is easier to reverse obesity in small and preteen children than in adolescents. This is because unhealthy lifestyles

have become habitual for a longer periods of time in obese adolescents than in obese children, and unhealthy lifestyles of longer duration are more difficult to reverse (Epstein et al. 1994, 373–383; Spear et al. 2007, S254–S288).

- Just because your obese child is an adolescent and her success rate is lower does not mean that your child should not try to control the weight. Many recent studies indicate that your obese adolescent child has a fair chance of succeeding (Barlow et al. 2007, S164–S192). The risk of not making the effort is too great.

The more risk factors for heart disease and diabetes your child has, the more urgent it is to institute immediate changes. Fortunately, obesity is a modifiable and correctable risk factor.

Approaches to Weight Control

Achieving a negative energy balance is the cornerstone of weight-management efforts. That means that you must ensure that your child consumes fewer calories by selecting healthy food while encouraging increased physical activity to expend more calories. A negative energy balance is achieved by practicing the 5-2-1-0 message and reducing SoFAS.

Reduce Calorie Intake

Overweight children should be placed on a balanced, lower-calorie diet by doing the following:

- Select food, fruits, and vegetables that are naturally low in fat and sugar and high in fiber and vitamins.
- Reduce or eliminate high-sugar drinks and snacks.
- Reduce consumption of high-fat foods such as French fries, chips, high-fat toppings on pizza (sausage, pepperoni, bacon, or extra cheese), and high-fat condiments (mayonnaise, cream-based sauces, regular sour cream, and regular salad dressing).
- Reduce the frequency of eating restaurant food, and have family dinners more often.
- Select lean meats, poultry, and fish.
- Make the home environment supportive of healthy eating, and do not keep high-fat and high-sugar snacks visible or accessible to children.

Be More Physically Active

Physical activity is an integral part of achieving a negative energy balance. Physical activities burn calories and help achieve negative energy balance. Without increasing physical activity and reducing sedentary lifestyle behavior, weight-control efforts do not succeed.

- Encourage your child to be play outside, weather permitting. Anything he or she does outside is better than spending time in front of a screen. Children should participate in some form of physical activity for more than an hour a day almost every day of the week, with more intense activity for thirty minutes three times per week.

- Reduce sedentary activities that do not burn many calories. The American Academy of Pediatrics (AAP) recommends that parents limit their child's screen time (i.e., TV, video games, and computer work) to no more than two hours per day (American Academy of Pediatrics 2000–2001).

What Are the Chances That Your Child Will Succeed?

By using the approaches in this book, the prospects of your child's success should be as good as using a professional weight-management program. Most weight-management clinics use protocols similar to those in this book. The following studies of parent-guided weight-management efforts offer further encouragement.

- Dr. Moria Golan and her colleagues in Israel published a noteworthy study in 1998 that is particularly helpful (Golan et al. 1998, 1130–1135). In a one-year study of obese children six to eleven years of age, the subjects were divided into two groups. In one group, the children were targeted with thirty hours of educational sessions. In the other group, only the parents of the children were targeted, with fourteen hours of instruction. The results were much better in the parent-only group than in the children-only group. In the parent-only group, 35 percent of obese children were no longer obese at the end of one year, while 79 percent of the children lost more than 10 percent of their relative weight. (Relative weight is expressed as a percentage of the ideal weight for the child's height, age, and gender. A 10 percent reduction in relative weight is considered successful weight control in adults and children.) These results are as good as many supervised weight-management clinics, and may even be better than some of them.

- An Australian study by Dr. Anthea Magarey and her coworkers in 2011 reported the effectiveness of parent-conducted weight-control efforts on preadolescent children five to nine years old (Margarey et al. 2011, 214–222). They reported an approximate 10 percent reduction in relative weight in six months, and the loss was maintained for at least two years without additional intervention.

The findings of these studies are encouraging for parents who are planning to help their overweight child. As indicated, the studies were carried out in preteen children. Similar studies involving adolescents are lacking, however. Though researchers have shown that the results of weight-control efforts in adolescents, in general, are not as good as in preteen children, many obese adolescents nonetheless succeed in weight control (Spear et al. 2007, S254–S288).

Success Rate of Weight-Control Efforts

The overall success rate of professionally supervised weight-management clinics is not as good as clinics that treat common medical problems such as ear infections, diarrhea, or asthma. Reasons why some children do not succeed in controlling their weight may include the following:

- One of the unique aspects of weight-management clinics is that doctors do not use medicine in the treatment of obesity (except for severe obesity). They rely on the motivation of the child and the support of the family.
- Some children (and their families) are not motivated to change their lifestyle. Although healthcare providers will provide advice and guidance to the child and family, ultimately it is the child who must change his lifestyle, and the degree of support the child receives from parents, family, and friends is critical to initiate and maintain motivation.
- Parental involvement is required to successfully change the child's lifestyle. Some parents who enroll their child in weight clinics are not motivated and do not actively participate in the process. They want to be involved only peripherally and rely on the expertise of the healthcare professionals. This lack of direct parental involvement increases the likelihood that weight-control efforts will fail.

Potential Advantages of Parent-Initiated Weight-Control Efforts

There are several reasons why you may achieve greater success than weight-management clinics:

- You are motivated to guide your child's lifestyle change. You are an active participant by your own decision. You are likely to become a role model for your child's healthy habits. This alone is a strong indication that you will succeed.
- You will be knowledgeable about weight-management techniques. By reading this book, you learn as much about weight management as you would if you were educated by weight-clinic staff. The book will function as a full-time, on-demand consultant.
- You will be a full-time counselor for your child rather than a part-time counselor at a weight clinic who sees your child briefly every one to four weeks. Because you are with your child every day, you are in a better position than counselors to educate your child and monitor your child's daily behavior.
- In addition to these advantages, parents themselves benefit. The knowledge and experience they gain in guiding their child through weight-control techniques frequently improves their own health. In a follow-up study, Dr. Golan and her associates found that parents in the parent-only group (discussed earlier) improved their eating habits, mothers lowered their LDL cholesterol, and fathers lost significant weight and lowered their glucose and triglyceride levels (Golan et al. 1999, 519–526). Take advantage of this occasion to improve your health and that of your family members.

Chapter 5

How to Make Lifestyle Changes

This chapter forms the core of healthy lifestyle change. All thirty lifestyle questions from chapter 3 are discussed, including unhealthy lifestyle behaviors that contribute to becoming overweight.

For each topic, the following are provided:

- Knowledge. Knowledge is provided with regard to scientific facts, how they may have contributed to obesity, and why unhealthy habits should be changed.
- Health goals. The section lists goals for healthy lifestyle change.
- Suggestions. These are practical strategies that you can use to make significant lifestyle changes. Additional material in chapter 10 is also suggested when appropriate.

Review your answers to the lifestyle questions in chapter 3, and identify those answers that are not consistent with a healthy lifestyle. Before you start, read this chapter to learn about the areas that you intend to change. You may want to read these topics selectively or read the whole chapter, depending on your plan of action. It is strongly advised that you read the entire chapter at some point, though, including the topics for which lifestyle changes are not needed.

While reading, think about how your child acquired his unhealthy habits. Some of them may be traced back to you. Revisit this chapter frequently. If you want in-depth information on certain topics, refer to chapter 10.

Physical Activity

How many days a week (on average) does your child play outside for at least sixty minutes? Include time spent at school in physical education (PE) class, organized and unorganized activities, and house chores.

Knowledge

- Insufficient physical activity (or inactivity, like TV watching) is one of the most important contributors to the development of obesity.
- Increasing physical activity is a critical component of all weight-control programs; diet or healthy eating alone does not work. One explanation for this may be that when one tries to lose weight by reducing caloric intake alone, the body goes into "starvation mode," drops its metabolic rate dramatically, and offsets the weight loss. It may be that a survival instinct kicks in when the body senses an inadequate supply of calories.
- Exercise not only burns calories but also tends to increase metabolic rate.
- The health benefits of physical activity include the following:

  a. Helps control weight
  b. Lowers LDL cholesterol and increases HDL cholesterol
  c. Reduces the risk of developing type 2 diabetes
  d. Lowers blood pressure
  e. Improves physical fitness
  f. Elevates mood
  g. Provides an opportunity to make friends

- Aerobic exercise is preferred. In general, aerobic exercise burns twice as many calories as weightlifting (for example). Examples of aerobic exercise include dancing, brisk walking, jogging, bicycling, swimming, ice- or roller-skating, and using aerobic gym equipment (e.g., treadmill or stationary bike).

Health Goals

- Children should be physically active for more than sixty minutes every day, as recommended by the AAP and other government agencies.
- Of the sixty minutes, at least thirty minutes should be spent in moderate activity that makes the child sweat and breathe heavily.

Suggestions

- Make simple, inexpensive equipment available to your child (e.g., bicycle, jump rope, or Frisbee). You do not need costly exercise equipment like a treadmill, and you do not have to enroll your child in a class with expensive sign-up fees.
- If starting an exercise program, start with activities of short duration and moderate intensity, and then gradually increase the duration and intensity.

- Some obese children may prefer exercising in a less structured setting that allows them to explore independently, such as free play, ice skating, Frisbee throwing, or bowling.
- Find activities that your child enjoys and are not too physically demanding. Your child may not be able to keep up with peers, and this may make him or her give up the effort. Emphasize fun, not winning or skill.
- Physical activity does not need to occur all at once; it can occur in several short sessions.
- Encourage children to be physically active during the day by walking to school or other nearby facilities or performing household chores like raking leaves and washing the car.
- Encourage your child to stay outside when the homework is done. Anything he or she does outside is better than watching TV or playing electronic games.
- Be a role model for your child, and exercise with your child as often as possible.
- Check what your child does during PE classes. Some schools do not use PE classes effectively and do not encourage children to be physically active.
- Plan activities for the whole family. When you are active together, your child will see how important exercise and staying fit are to you. These are activities that the family can do together:

    a. Play catch in the yard, or spend time hitting a tennis ball at the neighborhood courts.
    b. Take a hike or bike ride.
    c. Go to the park, and throw the football back and forth.
    d. Play tag in the front yard.
    e. Go to the community pool for a swim.
    f. Go to the mall, and walk from one end to the other (without spending time at the food court).
    g. Do household chores together such as cleaning, raking leaves, or waxing the car.

- Consider purchasing a pedometer (a device that measures the number of steps you take in a day), and set a starting goal of twelve thousand steps a day for your child. This is further discussed in chapter 10.

Screen Time

How many hours per day does your child watch TV/DVDs/videotapes, work on a computer, or play electronic games?

Knowledge

- Screen time refers to time spent watching TV and DVDs, working on computers, and playing electronic games. These sedentary activities are major contributors to the increasing prevalence of overweight and obese children.
- There is a strong association between overweight status and TV viewing in children. Reducing screen time is as important as increasing physical activity for successful weight management (Crespo et al. 2001, 360–365).
- Some children spend too much time on computers, especially surfing the Internet. It is estimated that about 10 percent of children are Internet addicted. (An "Internet addiction" is defined by compulsive Internet use for many hours, resulting in damage in areas such as social relationships, pleasurable physical activities, adequate sleep, schoolwork, or employment.) (Cash et al. 2012, 292–298.)
- How do watching TV and participating in other screen-time activities cause children to gain weight?

   a. They reduce time for other forms of physical activity that burn more energy.
   b. They may result in increased energy intake (due to snacking during viewing or in response to food commercials).
   c. They may reduce the body's resting metabolic rate (RMR).

- Other health-related and social problems associated with increased amounts of TV watching include lower school grades, attention deficit hyperactivity disorder (ADHD), decreased manual dexterity, and lower social development.

Health Goals

- Reduce screen time. The AAP recommends that screen time for children should be less than two hours a day.

Suggestions

- Parents should monitor the children's viewing habits and set a limit of less than two hours a day.
- Remove TVs from the child's bedroom (recommended by the AAP). Having a TV in a child's bedroom is associated with increased viewing.
- Do not put a computer in the child's room. Computers should be in an area of the home where parents can easily monitor what the child is doing.

CASE 1

KJ, a 10-year-old boy, was referred to the Weight Management Clinic for mild obesity. He weighed 52.8 kg (116 lb.) and measured 146 cm. (57.5 in.) tall. His BMI was 24.8, slightly above the 95th percentile (BMI =22.1). He lives in a small farming town outside a major city.

The lifestyle questionnaire showed that he watches TV from the time he comes home from school until dinner time. After dinner he continues to watch TV with the rest of the family. He eats a fairly balanced diet. The family almost never goes to fast food restaurants and they have a family dinner almost every day. They eat plenty of vegetables and grain products. The mother stocks enough sodas for her children so that they can have them anytime they want. She also keeps potato chips at home. However, KJ rarely eats the chip; they are mostly consumed by his dad when he drinks beer. KJ usually drinks 2 to 3 sodas a day. The family eats white bread and drinks whole milk.

During an educational session, the mother and KJ learned what they were doing was unhealthy. The main problems in this case were lack of physical activity (inactivity) due to too many hours watching TV and drinking too many high calorie sodas. KJ did not really like to watch TV but he had few out-of-school activities to participate in because the family lived in a small town. He did not particularly like to drink soda, but they were always available in the home. They also learned that one can of soda contain about 150 Calories and that KJ will have to walk briskly for a half hour or slowly for 1 hour to burn that many calories.

Three lifestyle change goals were prescribed: (1) to reduce TV watching time, (2) to reduce consumption of soda, and (3) to initiate an exercise program.

KJ's father arranged to have KJ's old bicycle repaired. KJ and his mother started riding their bicycles on a country road two miles every day, weather permitting. He reduced his television viewing. His mother stopped stocking sodas and KJ stopped drinking them without complaint. Having gained new knowledge about healthy eating, the family decided to switch from whole milk to 2 % milk and from white bread to whole wheat bread.

Within a month, KJ lost 8 lb. and grew 1 cm. which put his BMI (20.7) near the 90th percentile. He continued to make progress, and in 4 months he reduced his weight to the overweight range. At 1 year follow-up, his BMI was in the normal range.

This case illustrates how simple lack of knowledge about the causes of obesity can promote weight gain. Once KJ and his parents learned the causes of obesity, they stopped unhealthy behaviors with relatively little effort. Even with small changes in lifestyle, JK saw impressive rewards in as few as one month.

Whole-Grain Products

How many days in a week does your child eat whole-grain cereals, oatmeal, or other whole-grain products?

Knowledge

- In addition to fruits and vegetables, whole grains are an important source of fiber and other nutrients. Grain products should be a major component of a healthy diet (about a quarter of a plate, as shown in MyPlate).
- Grain products are divided into whole grain and refined grain. Whole-grain products are healthy, but refined-grain products are not.

    a. Whole grain refers to grain that contains three parts: endosperm, bran, and germ. (The structure of a grain is shown in fig. 10.3.) Bran, the outer layer, contains large amounts of fiber, B vitamins, and minerals. Germ, the embryo inside the seed, contains B vitamins, antioxidants, and phytochemicals that fight infection. Endosperm, the core, contains mostly carbohydrates (sugars) and some protein.

    b. Refined grain (like processed white flour) is mostly endosperm and lacks both bran and germ, which are removed during processing. White flour has not only a high glycemic index (GI) food, but also lacks fiber, vitamins, and minerals. This is why B vitamins and iron are frequently added back to white flour (referred to as "enriched"). This is why B vitamins and iron are frequently added back to white flour (referred to as "enriched"). GI is a measurement that rates foods on a scale from 1 to 100 based on the rate at which they raise blood sugar levels, with the GI of glucose set at 100. High GI foods are unhealthy. White flour products (with a high GI) raise blood sugar levels quickly and contribute to weight gain.

- The health benefits of consuming whole-grain products are as follows:

    a. They are low in fat and sugar and thus low in calories.
    b. They are low-GI food without the unhealthy consequences of high-GI foods. See the next section, Breads, for a brief discussion of GI, and see "Glycemic Index and Glycemic Load" in chapter 10 for a detailed discussion of the topic.
    c. They are a good source of dietary fiber and nutrients, such as folate, B vitamins, and minerals.

- Examples of whole-grain food include whole-grain breakfast cereals, whole-wheat and whole-grain breads, whole-grain pasta, whole-grain waffles, brown rice, popcorn, oats, and oatmeal.
- The 2010 dietary guidelines for Americans include the following:

    a. Persons age nine and older should eat three to five servings or more of whole grains every day. Consuming this amount of whole-grain products per day can reduce the risk of several chronic diseases and may help with weight control.

b. All Americans should make half or more of their grain products whole grain by replacing refined grains with whole grains. Many grain foods contain both whole grains and refined grains. As long as more than half of the food is whole grain, it is acceptable.

c. It is advisable to include folate-fortified products, such as folate-fortified whole-grain cereals, in whole-grain choices.

- Dietary fiber in whole-grain products provides a number of health benefits: proper bowel function, lowering cholesterol levels, reducing the risk of heart attacks and strokes, and preventing certain cancers. The recommended amount of dietary fiber for children is 1 g per year of age plus 5–10 g per day. For example, a six-year-old child should consume 6 g plus 5–10 g, which equals 11–16 g per day. For adults, 20–25 g per day is recommended. This topic is discussed further in "Dietary Fiber" in chapter 10.

Health Goals

- Eat whole-grain cereals and breads or other whole-grain products as often as possible.
- Eat at least 3 oz. of whole grain daily.

Suggestions

- Whole-grain cereals served with 1 percent or skim milk and topped with fruit is a healthy choice for breakfast. If your child does not eat cereal, choose other whole-grain products such as whole-grain bread. Do not serve sugary children's cereal.
- Some examples of ways to increase whole grain in the diet are as follows:

a. For breakfast, serve whole-grain bread, hot oatmeal, whole-grain breakfast cereal, a whole-grain muffin, or a whole-grain bagel.

b. Use 100 percent whole-wheat bread to make sandwiches.

c. When baking, replace one-third of white flour with whole-wheat flour or oatmeal.

d. Add brown rice to recipes instead of white rice or use whole-grain pasta instead of regular pasta.

e. Popcorn is a whole grain.

- You can find whole-grain foods when shopping:

a. The percent daily value (percent DV) for fiber found on the food label is a good clue as to the amount of whole grain in the product.

b. Color is not an indication of a whole grain. Bread can be brown due to a dye or molasses.

c. Check the ingredient lists on food labels, and make sure that whole wheat, whole grain, brown rice, oats, or oatmeal are listed as the main ingredient. (Food contents are listed in descending order of amount.) Words like "enriched

(Continues at the bottom of the next page)

Breads

What kind of bread does your child eat at home?

Knowledge

- White bread is a high-GI food. After eating one slice of white bread, blood glucose level rises as high and as quickly as after eating a teaspoonful of table sugar. A quick and high rise in blood glucose has unhealthy consequences. GI has become an important concept in developing an understanding of obesity, as discussed in "Glycemic Index and Glycemic Load" in chapter 10.
- Most starchy foods, chiefly those made out of refined grain and potatoes, have a high GI. Sugar-sweetened foods like cookies, candies, muffins, soft drinks, sugar-coated cereals, instant rice, cornflakes, and honey also have a high GI.
- In contrast, whole-wheat bread is a low-GI food and contains dietary fiber, vitamins, and minerals. Switching from white bread to whole-wheat bread has been shown to reduce the risk of heart disease by 20 percent in adults.
- High-GI foods (including white breads) are unhealthy for several reasons:

    a. They raise blood levels of sugar and insulin quickly to a high level. High levels of insulin drive not only glucose in the blood into body cells but also drive blood lipids into body cells, resulting in fat accumulation (or weight gain).

    b. They raise triglyceride levels in blood, which is a known risk factor for heart disease. The mechanism of how high-GI foods raise triglyceride levels is discussed in "High Triglyceride Levels" in chapter 10.

    c. The feeling of satiety is shorter after eating a high-GI food, and one ends up overeating, contributing to weight gain.

    d. They are usually low in dietary fiber, vitamins, minerals, and other nutrients.

Health Goals

- Reduce consumption of white bread and breads made from enriched flour.
- Switch to whole-wheat or other whole-grain breads.

Suggestions

- Serve whole-wheat bread for all meals instead of white bread.
- Read "Glycemic Index and Glycemic Load" and "High Triglyceride Levels" in chapter 10.

Whole Grain (Continued.)

flour," "degerminated," "bran," or "wheat germ" indicate that the product is not whole grain.

- Read "Grain Group of Food," "Glycemic Index and Glycemic Load," "Dietary Fiber," and "More on MyPlate" in chapter 10.

Potatoes

How many days a week does your child eat potatoes (such as baked potatoes, mashed potato, or potato salad) as the main portion of a meal?

Knowledge

- Although potatoes are vegetables, unlike other common vegetables they contain large amounts of starch. Thus, potato is not a recommended variety of vegetable.
- Consumption of large amounts of potatoes is unhealthy because of the following:

    a. Potatoes are a high-GI food (which raises blood sugar and insulin to a high level) with consequent weight gain as discussed under the headline "Breads." Research has shown a positive association between intake of potatoes and weight gain among adults (Mozaffarian et al. 2011, 1901–1613).
    b. They do not contain much dietary fiber. Only the skin of the potato has fiber.

- French fries are doubly unhealthy, because they are also high in fat and calories and can raise blood cholesterol.
- Potato chips are worse than French fries, because they are high in fat and sodium. They are deep-fried in oil and seasoned with salt. Excessive consumption of potato chips is one of the most important contributors to weight change. High sodium intake may cause high blood pressure (hypertension).

Health Goals

- Avoid excessive consumption of potatoes, and eat more green leafy vegetables.

Suggestions

- Choose green leafy vegetables instead of starchy vegetables like potatoes.
- Reduce consumption of other potato products such as French fries, potato chips, and breads made from potato flour.
- Read "Glycemic Index and Glycemic Load" and "Dietary Fiber" in chapter 10.

Fruits and Vegetables

How many days a week does your child eat at least 1½ cups of fruit (2 cups for adolescents)?

How many days a week does your child eat at least 2½ cups of vegetables, such as green, yellow, orange, or red vegetables (3 cups for adolescents)? Do not include potatoes.

Knowledge

- Americans consume too few servings of fruits and vegetables. MyPlate recommends that half the plate be fruits and vegetables. Increasing consumption of fruits and vegetables will reduce the consumption of high-fat, high-calorie food, thus helping to reduce calories taken in and control weight.
- There are numerous health benefits from eating fruits and vegetables:

  a. They are low in calories, make you feel full sooner, and their consumption delays further hunger. Thus they prevent you from taking in excess calories.
  b. They are associated with decreased risk of developing diabetes, heart disease, stroke, and certain types of cancers.
  c. They are high in fiber, which helps regulate bowel movement and lowers blood cholesterol.
  d. Most fruits are excellent sources of vitamins A and C.
  e. They are high in potassium, which helps to lower blood pressure.

Health Goals

- Eat at least five servings of fruits and vegetables a day.
- Even better, eat more than 1½ cups of fruits and more than 2½ cups of vegetables each day (½ cup more for adolescents and adults).
- Fill half of your food plate with fruits and vegetables (as seen in MyPlate).

Suggestions

- All fresh, canned, dried, and frozen fruits and vegetables are good options.
- Avoid fruits and vegetables that are prepared with high-fat ingredients (French fries, vegetables cooked in cheese or cream sauces, vegetables served with added bacon or butter, fruit pies, or fruit served with whipped cream).
- Remember and practice the 5-2-1-0 message.
- Here are some tips to help your child and family eat more fruit:

  a. At breakfast, top your cereal with bananas or peaches. Add blueberries to pancakes, or try fruit mixed with low-fat or fat-free yogurt.
  b. For lunch, pack a tangerine, banana, or grapes, or choose fruits from a salad bar.
  c. At dinner, add crushed pineapple to coleslaw, or include mandarin oranges or grapes in a tossed salad.
  d. For dessert, have fresh or baked apples, pears, or a fruit salad.

e. Keep a bowl of fresh fruit in the refrigerator at eye level. Sliced or cut fruit makes a great snack. Try whole, fresh berries or grapes.

f. Dried fruits make a great snack. They are easy to carry and store. Examples include apricots, apples, pineapples, bananas, cherries, figs, dates, cranberries, blueberries, prunes (dried plums), and raisins. Note that sulfur dioxide (SO_2) is used as an antioxidant in some dried fruits to protect their color and flavor, which can induce asthma when inhaled or ingested by sensitive people. About 1 percent of healthy people and 5 percent of patients with asthma are estimated to be sensitive to sulfite.

g. Frozen juice bars (100 percent juice) make healthy alternatives to high-fat snacks.

h. Fruit juices are not as good as fruit itself, though, because they contain less dietary fiber than whole fruit.

- Here is a list of suggestions to help your child and family eat more vegetables:

a. Plan main meals around a vegetable, such as a vegetable stir-fry or soup.

b. Shred carrots or zucchini into meatloaf, casseroles, quick breads, and muffins.

c. Include chopped vegetables in pasta sauce or lasagna.

d. Grill vegetable kabobs as part of a barbecue meal. Try tomatoes, mushrooms, green pepper, spinach, or onions.

e. Prepare a soup that contains vegetables, such as minestrone.

f. Serve a lettuce salad with your dinner several times every week.

g. Add lettuce, tomato, green pepper, spinach, or onion to sandwiches.

h. Keep a bowl of cut vegetables in a clear container in the refrigerator; children may reach for them.

i. Vary your vegetable choices to keep meals interesting.

j. Involve children in shopping and food preparation. Children can help shop for, clean, peel, or cut vegetables. While shopping, allow children to pick out a new vegetable to try at home.

k. There are many websites containing recipes for main and side dishes using vegetables. A few are listed here:

- 386 results for vegetable dish (by Victor Chang):
  http://www.cooks.com/rec/search/0,1-0, vegetable_dish, FF.html
- 10 vegetable main dishes (Mayo clinic):
  http://www.mayoclinic.com/health/food-and nutrition?NU00203
- Vegetable salad recipe:
  http://allrecipes.com/Recipes/salad/vegetable-salads/main.aspx

- Read "Fruits and Vegetables" and "Energy Density" in chapter 10.

Snacks

How many days a week does your child eat vegetables (not potatoes) or sliced fruits as a snack?

Knowledge

- As a general guideline, children should have two snacks a day, preferably low-calorie food such as fruits and vegetables. Some children eat too many snacks.
- Eating high-fat, high-calorie snacks results in extra calorie intake and contributes to weight gain. Examples of unhealthy snacks include potato chips, cookies, candy, French fries, and pizza.
- Examples of healthy alternatives include carrots or celery sticks, a cup of melon or strawberries, a cup of light microwave popcorn, an apple, a cup of vegetable soup, sugar-free gelatin, and fruit snacks.

Health Goals

- Make snacks with fruits and vegetables the norm.
- Avoid unhealthy snacks such as cookies, donuts, potato chips, and soft drinks.

Suggestions

- Have fruits and vegetables available in the house and accessible to your child at all times. Allow your child to have as many fruit and vegetable snacks as she wants.
- Do not buy unhealthy, fatty, or sweet snacks. If they are in the house, make them less visible or inaccessible to your child.
- Read "Fruits and Vegetables" and "Energy Density" in chapter 10.

Milk

What type of milk does your child drink?

Knowledge

- Milk is a good source of protein. It is also a good source of calcium and vitamin D, which are important for healthy bone building. Children older than two years are encouraged to drink at least 2 cups of milk each day. Milk contains saturated fat, which can raise blood cholesterol levels and add calories.

- Although skim, 1 percent, and 2 percent milks have a lower fat and calorie content, they contain the nutrients that are present in whole milk, such as calcium and vitamin D.

- Whole milk has 3.25 percent fat and provides 150 Calories per 8 oz. (or 1 cup). Two percent milk has 120 Calories. One percent milk has 100 Calories, and skim milk has 80 Calories in the same volume. If your child drinks 3 cups of milk a day, switching to 1 percent or skim milk will reduce her calorie intake by 150 or 210 Calories a day.

- Chocolate milk is a high-sugar drink with more calories than whole milk or sodas. It provides 200 Calories and contains 30 g sugar per 8 oz.

- Soy milk (Silk brand) provides 100 Calories per 8 oz., similar to 1 percent milk.

Health Goals

- Use skim or 1 percent milk instead of whole milk for children over two years of age.

Suggestions

- Buy 1 percent or skim milk instead of whole milk.
- If children resist switching from whole milk to 1 percent or skim milk, this can be done gradually by mixing increasingly smaller amounts of the higher-fat milk with the lower-fat milk.
- Read "Good Fats and Bad Fats" in chapter 10.

Cheeses

How many days a week does your child eat American, cheddar, Swiss, or Monterey Jack cheese instead of low-fat or part-skim cheese for a snack or on sandwiches or pizza?

Knowledge

- Cheese is a wonderful source of protein and calcium, but it is also a major source of saturated fat and sodium. Saturated fat raises blood cholesterol levels, and sodium raises blood pressure. Too much of either is unhealthy. Americans are heavy users of cheese, especially on pizza and hamburgers.
- The fat content of cheeses varies:
  a. Regular cheeses provide 8 to 9 g of fat per ounce.
  b. Reduced-fat cheeses have about 6 g of fat per ounce.
  c. Low-fat cheeses have 3 g or less fat per ounce.

- The fat and calorie content of cheeses varies:
  a. Regular American, blue, cheddar, and Swiss cheeses are high in fat (> 100 Calories per ounce).
  b. Part-skim mozzarella, string cheese, farmer's cheese, and Neufchâtel are naturally low in fat (70–85 Calories per ounce).
  c. Reduced-fat cheeses are widely available, such as cheddar, Monterey Jack, mozzarella, Brie, Swiss, colby, Muenster, and American.

- The sodium content of cheeses varies:
  a. American, blue, and parmesan cheeses have a high sodium content (approximately 400 mg sodium per ounce).
  b. Cheddar, mozzarella, and cottage cheeses have a medium sodium content (approximately 130–180 mg).
  c. Swiss cheese has a much lower sodium content (less than 60 mg per ounce).

Health Goals

- Use low- or reduced-fat cheese instead of regular cheese.

Suggestions

- Use cheese in moderation.
- Use low-fat cheese instead of regular cheese to reduce intake of fat and calories.
- Choose low-sodium cheese (such as Swiss, cheddar, mozzarella) over high-sodium cheese (like American, blue, and parmesan).
- Part-skim mozzarella is one of the best choices, because it is low in calories, saturated fat, and sodium (72 Cal, 4–5 g of fat, and 175 mg sodium per ounce).
- While grocery shopping, check the nutrition facts label for the amount of saturated fat as well as the sodium content.
- At restaurants, choose hamburgers over cheeseburgers, and use cheese toppings in moderation.
- Read "Excessive Salt Intake" and "Good Fats and Bad Fats" in chapter 10.

Burgers (and School Lunches)

How many times a week does your child eat hamburgers or cheeseburgers? Include those eaten at the school cafeteria.

Knowledge

- A typical American fast-food meal includes a hamburger or cheeseburger, French fries, and a soft drink, all of which are high in fat and sugar and therefore high in calories. Although smaller portions of fast food may supply about 650 Calories, larger servings can add up to 1,300 Calories or more, which is more than half of the daily calorie allowance for children.

- Research has shown that the frequency of consumption of fast food with soft drinks is positively related to the prevalence of obesity and other diseases like type 2 diabetes and heart disease (Bowman et al. 2004, 112–118; Thompson et al. 2004, 282–289).

- Fast foods are unhealthy because of the following:

  a. They are usually high in fat, sugar, and calories.
  b. They are low in fiber and vitamins.
  c. Large servings of soft drinks add significant calories.

- Hamburgers are a key item in fast food and are an essential part of American cuisine. They are popular among children and widely available in school cafeterias. They are often served with bacon, lettuce, tomatoes, cheese, onions, and pickles. Additions such as ketchup, mustard, and mayonnaise add to the taste but also add calories. Quarter-pound hamburgers may total a whopping 459 Calories.

- Cheeseburgers are popular among Americans. One slice of cheese on a cheeseburger adds 8–10 g of fat (about 100 Calories).

School Cafeteria Food

- An overwhelming 94 percent of American schools participate in the National School Lunch Program, and twenty-one million students relied on school lunches as their main meal in 2012.

- Many school cafeteria foods are more similar to fast food than you might think. Hamburgers, cheeseburgers, and French fries are popular items. The government estimates that two-thirds of school meals exceed the allowable amount of fat (Center for Disease Control and Prevention. December 2009). Most have too much sodium and are low in fiber.

- Some school cafeterias offer healthy foods including fruits, vegetables, and salad, but the problem is that children don't eat them. Children are not aware of the healthful nature of fruits and vegetables and are not used to eating them.

- The school lunch guidelines (announced in January 2011 by the USDA) are expected to improve the quality of school cafeteria food. All K–12 public schools must start serving school lunches according to the new guidelines, which are being implemented gradually. When fully implemented, the new school lunch guidelines will achieve the following:

a. Establish the first calorie limits for school meals
b. Gradually reduce the amount of sodium by more than half over ten years
c. Ban most trans fats
d. Require more servings of fruits and vegetables
e. Require milk to be low fat or nonfat, and require flavored milks (like chocolate milk) to be nonfat
f. Increase the amount of whole grains, eventually requiring that most grains are whole grain
g. Limit students to 1 cup of starchy vegetables a week, meaning schools will not be able to offer French fries every day

- Even with the implementation of this program, some cafeteria foods remain unhealthy, according to a 2014 report from the University of Michigan Health System. The report found that two out of three middle school students who eat school lunches regularly are overweight or obese. In addition, they may have higher LDL cholesterol than kids who bring their lunch. Students who eat a school lunch regularly are less likely to eat two servings of fruits and vegetables each, more likely to drink sugary drinks, and less likely to participate in school sports activities (WebMD News Archive. March 15, 2010).

Health Goals
- Limit the consumption of hamburgers and cheeseburgers.

Suggestions
- Reduce the number of meals consisting of fast food and "junk food" (food that is of little nutritional value). It is often high in fat, sugar, salt, and calories with little protein, vitamins, or minerals. Examples of junk food include salted snacks, candy, sweet desserts, fried fast food, and sugary carbonated drinks.
- Check the school cafeteria menu, and choose healthy foods with your child. Follow up to make sure that your child is choosing and eating the healthy choices.
- You may want to pack your child a healthy lunch if you find the school cafeteria lunch to be unhealthy. A grilled chicken or turkey breast on whole-wheat bread is a healthy choice. Add a piece of fruit and a small bottle of water, or encourage the child to buy low-fat milk in the cafeteria. Do not pack potato chips, cookies, breakfast bars, and so on.
- Read "Good Fats and Bad Fats" and "How to Reduce Fat Intake" in chapter 10.

CASE 2

AM, a 14-year-old female, was referred to the Weight Management Clinic for moderate obesity. Her BMI 32.2 was higher than the 95th percentile, between the 95th and the 99th percentile lines.

AM's lifestyle questionnaire showed that she watches TV from the time she comes home from school until dinner time. After dinner she continues to watch TV with the rest of the family. She lives in an apartment complex in a big city. Both of her parents work. She does not like to play with neighborhood friends. She eats school lunch every day and her favorite meal choice is a cheeseburger with French fries. On weekends, her family eats at fast food restaurants because her mother is too tired to cook. Everybody in the family likes to drink soda and fruit drinks. Her mother keeps potato chips stocked at home all the time. AM occasionally eats chips while watching TV. The family eats white bread and drinks whole milk regularly.

During the educational session at the Weight Management clinic, AM did not pay much attention and her mother did not seem to understand the gravity of her daughter's weight problem.

Three lifestyle change goals were recommended: (1) to reduce TV watching to no more than 4 hours a day; and (2) to go outside the house and do whatever she feels like doing for at least one hour every day; and (3) to reduce consumption of sugary drinks to no more than one bottle a day. The family reluctantly decided to change to 2 % milk but continued to eat white bread.

On her 1 month visit, AM had gained 4 lb. and was not keeping up with her recommended goals. At that visit, additional information became available. Her recent blood cholesterol level was slightly elevated (up to 220 mg./dL.) and her father, aged 46 years, was told he may have to have a bypass surgery for coronary artery disease. AM and her mother were told about the close relationship between cholesterol level and the father's heart problem. It turned out that her grandparents also experienced heart attacks at relatively young ages and her grandfather passed away in his 50s. AM and her mother seemed to grasp the gravity of her high cholesterol level, which they understood was caused by her being obese.

When AM returned to the clinic a month later, she had not gained any weight and she seemed to be trying to increase her physical activity level. One month later, she had lost 4 lb. and appeared very happy about what she had accomplished.

This case illustrates how providing information about the cardiovascular risk factors can serve as a wake-up call for AM to take her obesity seriously. Although she has not been able to lower her BMI to the overweight range, AM's cholesterol has decreased below 200 mg./dL. and she was more interested in changing her unhealthy lifestyle.

French Fries

How many times a week does your child eat French fries, hash browns, or tater tots? Include those eaten at the school cafeteria.

Knowledge

- French fries, hash browns, and tater tots are made of potatoes that have been deep-fried. Hash browns and tater tots absorb more fat during frying than French fries. These foods contain large amounts of fat, calories, and salt.

- It is estimated that Americans eat an average of four servings of French fries every week. Frequent consumption of French fries (and their variants) contributes to poor health for the following reasons:

  a. They are high in calories due to the high fat content from deep-frying, thereby contributing to weight gain. How many Calories are there in McDonald's French fries? A small container (2.5 oz.) has 230 Calories and 160 mg of sodium, and a large one (5.4 oz.) has 500 Calories and 350 mg of sodium.

  b. Although the use of trans fat in frying has decreased in recent years, consumption of trans fat is still a cause of heart disease. A recent study involving eighty thousand women showed that for every 5 percent increase in saturated fat in the diet, the prevalence of heart disease increased by 17 percent. However, for an extra 2 percent increase in trans fat, there was an extra 93 percent increase in the incidence of heart disease (Mozaffarian et al. 2006, 1601–1613).

  c. French fries are made from a high-GI carbohydrate, which is known to contribute to weight gain. This quickly absorbed carbohydrate is converted to glycogen, which can be stored in the body as fat.

  d. Acrylamide, a cancer-promoting substance in laboratory animals, is produced by frying potatoes.

- The salt content of French fries varies widely from restaurant to restaurant, with a large portion of French fries containing some 350–940 mg of sodium. Compare these numbers with the daily allowance of 2,400 mg. (Note that the daily allowance of sodium is 1,500 mg according to the dietary guidelines of 2010.)

- French fries are cooked in saturated fat from animals, such as beef tallow or lard, hydrogenated vegetable oil, or unsaturated vegetable oils. Both saturated fat and trans fat tend to increase LDL cholesterol and decrease HDL cholesterol. Trans fat is much worse than saturated fat for heart health. In recent years, many restaurants advertised the use of vegetable oils. Hydrogenation converts liquid vegetable oils to solid or semisolid fats (trans fat), which improves texture and shelf life. However, increased intake of trans fats was found to be more than ten times worse than saturated fat in increasing the risk of heart disease in women (Mozaffarian et al. 2006, 1601–1613). Foods like French fries, donuts, shortening, potato chips, and margarine have large amounts of trans fat. Although unsaturated vegetable oils do not raise LDL cholesterol, they provide significant amounts of calories.

- Acrylamide is formed when starch-rich foods are fried, baked, grilled, toasted, or microwaved at high temperatures. It is present in many foods regularly consumed in the world. French fries and potato chips are recognized as the two biggest sources of acrylamide in the American diet. Acrylamide is known to be a cancer-causing agent (a carcinogen) in laboratory animals. It is also suspected to be genotoxic, meaning that it can cause damage to the genetic material of cells. According to some studies, French fries and potato chips contain about three hundred times more acrylamide than the safety limits recommended by the World Health Organization (WHO) (National Cancer Institute. July 29, 2008). As of 2014, acrylamide is still in debate for its carcinogenicity links in humans. In the meantime, it would be wise to limit the intake of food containing acrylamide.

Health Goals
- Reduce the consumption of French fries, hash browns, tater tots, and similar foods.

Suggestions
- French fries are a key element of fast food, and reducing consumption of fast food or the frequency of eating out helps to reduce the intake of French fries.
- For adults and children, it is easy to take five minutes in the morning to pack healthier alternatives rather than eat fast food or restaurant food. This will save you money and keep you healthy.
- Read "Excessive Salt Intake" and "Good Fats and Bad Fats" in chapter 10.
- Learn how to choose healthy fast food by reading "How to Reduce Fat Intake" in chapter 10.

Fried Food

How many times a week does your child eat fried food (such as fried chicken, fried fish, etc.)?

Knowledge

- Fried food is not just French fries, fried chicken, and fried fish. Any vegetable or meat can be deep-fried (onion rings, sweet potato, steak, chicken, etc.).
- Many fried foods are not hot and greasy when presented (potato chips, corn chips, crackers, donuts, Twinkies, etc.).
- Fried foods are unhealthy because of the following:

  a. They are high in fat and calories. They cause weight gain and raise blood cholesterol, which in turn increases the risk of heart disease.
  b. Some of them can contain trans fats, which put you at a higher risk of heart disease.
  c. Foods such as donuts are also high in sugar, further increasing calories.
  d. Foods such as chips have a high salt content, which contributes to high blood pressure and risk of stroke.
  e. They are low in fiber. A deficiency of fiber may cause poor digestive function, increased risk of heart disease, and some types of cancers.

Health Goals

- Reduce consumption of all fried foods that are high in calories.

Suggestions

- Choose food that is baked, boiled, broiled, or steamed.
- Limit consumption of fried foods as well as potato chips, corn chips, crackers, and donuts.
- When cooking, do not deep-fry or pan-fry food; sautéing and stir-frying add much smaller amounts of fat. Read "Frying Food" in this chapter for cooking methods using fat.
- Use nonstick vegetable oil cooking spray instead of liquid oil.
- Read "Good Fats and Bad Fats" in chapter 10.

Chips

How many times a week does your child eat potato and other kinds of chips?

Knowledge

- The potato chip is the most popular snack in America. The global potato chip market accounted for 36 percent of the total snack market in 2005 ($46 billion).

- Potato chips (and other chips, including corn and tortilla chips) are produced by deep-frying in vegetable oil or saturated fat, and thus they are high in fat content. Some of them are high in trans fat as well, although many companies no longer deep-fry them in trans fat.

- Potato chips are unhealthy because of the following:

  a. High levels of fat and calories contribute to weight gain and obesity. Potato chips are a major contributor to the epidemic of obesity and have had a greater negative effect than consumption of potatoes and soft drinks.
  b. High saturated fat contents contribute to high cholesterol levels. Some chips have significant amounts of trans fats, which is worse than saturated fat in raising blood cholesterol levels and increasing risk of developing heart disease.
  c. Chips are typically low in vitamins and minerals.
  d. The high salt content is a major culprit in hypertension, which can lead to stroke, heart failure, and kidney disease.
  e. The health concerns of acrylamide in chips remain.

- One ounce of most types of potato chips (which is 11–18 chips) provides about 150 Calories and 160 mg sodium. Compare this to 150 Calories in a 12 oz. soda. Potato chips frequently come in large-sized bags, promoting increased consumption. The average size of the potato chip package has increased to about 14 oz., and people end up eating significantly more than the standard 1 oz. serving. The smallest individual packages contain 1 or 1.5 oz. Because most people eat more than 1 oz., the calorie and sodium intake become unacceptably high.

- Chips come in various flavors and seasonings, such as cheese, onion, vinegar, barbecue, and others.

- Baked chips are low in fat. The sodium content varies.

Health Goals

- Reduce consumption of chips (such as potato chips and corn chips).

Suggestions

- Reduce the frequency and amount of chip consumption.
- Baked chips are better choices than regular fried chips.
- Read "Excessive Salt Intake" and "Good Fats and Bad Fats" in chapter 10.

Sweet Food

How many times a day does your child eat sweet food (cakes, pies, ice cream, cookies, pastries, donuts, muffins, chocolate, or candy)?

Knowledge

- Sweet foods and sugary drinks provide "empty calories." These are foods that are high in calories but devoid of fiber, vitamins, and minerals, resulting in weight gain.
- Consumption of too much sugar is unhealthy for the following reasons:

    a. Excessive amounts of sugar elevate blood sugar (glucose) and insulin for longer-than-normal periods. Insulin promotes the movement of glucose from the circulation into the cells, and it allows circulating fat to enter fat cells, resulting in fat accumulation (weight gain).
    b. Sugar raises triglyceride levels, which can cause heart disease.
    c. Sweet foods lack important nutrients, vitamins, minerals, fiber, and protein.
    d. Sugar suppresses your appetite for more nourishing food and may actually increase hunger.
    e. Sugar promotes tooth decay.

- According to the WHO, the daily sugar allowance is 10 percent of total calories. For a ten-year-old who consumes 2,000 Calories per day, the daily allowance is 200 Calories or 50 g. The daily sugar allowance is 75 g for adolescents who take in 3,000 Calories a day. Compare this amount with 40 g of sugar in a 12 oz. can of Coca-Cola. This is nearly an entire day's allowance of sugar for a child.

Health Goals

- Reduce consumption of high-sugar foods.

Suggestions

- Make it a habit to choose food with low sugar content by reading the food label. Avoid buying food with more than 20 g of sugar per serving, which is 40 percent of the daily allowance. A sugar content of 10 g or less per serving is better.
- Reduce purchases of sodas, fruit drinks or punches, cakes, cookies, ice cream, and so forth.
- Substitute fruits and vegetables for sweets at snack time. Do not make sugary food accessible to children in the house.
- For dessert, serve fruit instead of conventional desserts such as pie, cake, or ice cream.
- When cooking, use less sugar than the recipe calls for.
- If you use canned fruit, drain the syrup before serving.
- During holidays, ration candy and other high-sugar (or high-fat) treats, and throw away the excess after one week.
- Read "Excessive Sugar Intake" in chapter 10.

Sodas

How many regular sodas does your child consume each day?

Knowledge

- Soft drinks account for 33 percent of the sugar intake among Americans. This is followed by sugar from candy (16 percent), cakes, cookies, and pies (13 percent), fruit drinks (10 percent), dairy dessert and milk products (9 percent), and others (6 percent). Sodas and other sugary drinks combined account for nearly half of the added sugars in the American diet and have contributed to the epidemic of obesity.

- Excessive consumption of soft drinks results in adverse health effects such as the following:

   a. They provide a large number of calories. There is evidence that consumption of soft drinks is directly related to weight gain (Troiano et al. 2000, 1343S–1353S).
   b. That weight gain, in turn, is a prime risk factor for type 2 diabetes, which, for the first time, is a problem for teens as well as adults.
   c. They are a problem because they have displaced milk and water.
   d. They provide energy but lack nutrients like vitamins, fiber, protein, and minerals.
   e. They may cause dental decay.
   f. They may be linked to hyperactivity disorders.
   g. Caffeine in soft drinks, taken within three hours of sleep, may cause disruption of sleep patterns and leave children feeling tired the following day. A 12 oz. soft drink has about 35 mg of caffeine; compare this with 100 mg of caffeine in 8 oz. of coffee. The AAP recommends that adolescents get no more than 100 mg of caffeine a day.
   h. They may increase the risk of osteoporosis. Phosphoric acid in the drink may displace calcium from bone.

- A single can of soda contains the equivalent of 10 teaspoons of sugar. Would you give your child a large glass of water that has 10 teaspoons of sugar in it? Would you drink it yourself? Would you allow your child to drink this every day and more than once every day? This amount of sugar, which is a high-GI food, especially in liquid form, makes blood sugar skyrocket and causes sustained elevation of insulin levels (hyperinsulinemia). Over time, this can lead to diabetes or insulin resistance, not to mention weight gain and other health problems.

- As discussed previously, the daily allowance of sugar is 50 g for a ten-year-old child (12.5 teaspoons) and 75 g (19 teaspoons) for an adolescent boy. A 12 oz. cola drink has about 40 g of sugar, which is about 80 percent of the daily sugar allowance, illustrating how easy it is to exceed the daily allowance.

- What do you have to do to burn the calories in a 12 oz. can of soda? A child weighing 130 lb. needs to walk slowly for one hour to burn 150 Calories, while uphill walking or walking very briskly for thirty minutes also burns 150 Calories.

- The following arithmetic shows how easy it is to gain weight by overconsumption of sodas and sugary drinks. It is estimated that 3,500 unused Calories become 1 lb. of fat; this is equivalent to the unburned calories from twenty-three cans of soda.
- Although not completely proved, high-fructose corn syrup in soft drinks has been blamed for having a major role in the detrimental effects of sugar. A number of studies have reported that fructose may cause metabolic syndrome and hypertriglyceridemia and lower the levels of HDL cholesterol, fatty liver, and so on. However, other studies, some of which have been supported by the beverage industry, dispute the claims (Kelishadi et al. 2014, 503–510).

Health Goal
- Reduce consumption of sodas as much as possible. Water is the best drink. Practice the 5-2-1-0 message, and consume no sugary drinks.

Suggestions
- Research done in Belgium has concluded that the following parenting practices may play an important role in reducing soda consumption (in decreasing order of importance) (Van der Horst et al. 2006, 295–304):

  a. Not offering soda at meal time
  b. Not letting kids drink soda whenever they want
  c. Not keeping soda in the house

- A simple approach is not buying sodas and not keeping them in the house. When available, children will reach for them.
- Make water and low-fat milk the drink of choice for all members of the family. Water is the best drink when you are thirsty.
- Diet sodas are acceptable only while transitioning to making water the primary drink. There is evidence that diet drinks (with saccharin and other artificial sweeteners) result in increased intake of calories and weight gain in laboratory rats (Fowler et al. 2008, 1894–1900).
- Read "Excessive Sugar Intake" in chapter 10.

Other Sugary Drinks

How many glasses of 100 percent fruit juice (such as orange juice) does your child drink in a day?

How many glasses of fruit drinks or fruit juice cocktails (Sunny Delight, Hi-C, Hawaiian Punch, lemonade, and other fruit-flavored drinks) does your child drink in a day?

Knowledge

- Fruit-flavored drinks (labeled "ade," punch, cocktail, etc.) do not contain much actual juice; they are made mostly of sugar and water.
- Both 100 percent fruit juices and fruit drinks (or punches) have large amounts of sugar.

  a. One hundred percent fruit juices such as orange juice, apple juice, and grape juice all have about 110 to 120 Calories in 8 oz. (compared to 100 Calories in Coca-Cola of the same volume).
  b. Most fruit drinks (or fruit cocktails) have as much or more sugar as regular sodas. Ocean Spray cranberry, Capri-Sun fruit drink, Minute Maid juice beverage, and Sunny Delight all have the sugar content of sodas.

- The AAP has recommended limiting consumption of 100 percent fruit juices, including orange juice, to 4–6 oz. per day for children one to six years of age and 8–12 oz. for children seven to eighteen years of age.
- Some "energy drinks" contain high amounts of sugar and 110–125 Calories in 8 oz. In addition, they contain stimulants like caffeine and taurine, which could cause agitation, irritability, insomnia, and heart rhythm problems.
- "Sports drinks" (Gatorade, Powerade, Allsport, etc.) supply optimal amounts of carbohydrates and electrolytes. They help prevent dehydration and restore minerals lost through perspiration after exercise. However, they should only be consumed after an extended period of hard exercise (more than one hour).

Health Goals

- Limit 100 percent fruit juices, including orange juice, to 6 oz. per day for children and 12 oz. per day for adolescents.
- Reduce consumption of fruit drinks or fruit cocktails.

Suggestions

- Limit consumption of 100 percent fruit juices. Instead, encourage children to eat whole fruits to meet the recommended daily fruit intake (1½ to 2 cups a day). Whole fruits have dietary fiber and other nutrients that may be lost in fruit juices.
- Do not buy fruit drinks or keep them in the house.
- Read "Excessive Sugar Intake" and "Energy Drinks and Sports Drinks" in chapter 10.

Portion Size

How much food does your child eat at each meal compared to his/her peers?

Knowledge

- If you think your child's portion size is large, this is not surprising. Americans tend to eat larger portions than people do in other countries. Portion sizes of popular dishes are 25 percent larger in the United States than in France, for example, where rates of obesity are lower.

- What could be the cause of larger portion sizes in America? It may have something to do with the large portion size of foods served in restaurants, especially fast-food outlets, and the increased frequency of people eating restaurant food. Many fast-food restaurants have "supersized" menu items. With an increased frequency of eating out, consumers are exposed to larger portions of food and have gotten used to consuming them.

- In weight-control efforts, the bottom line is total calorie intake. You can reduce total calorie intake by reducing portion size and/or consuming low-energy-density food (defined as food with a low value of calories per unit of weight or volume). Between these options, reducing portion size is more difficult. Simply advising someone "to eat less" may not be effective. Your hungry, overweight child is not going to listen to your command to "eat less." It is better to serve low-energy-density food such as fruits, vegetables, and whole-grain products while maintaining food volume or weight than to try to reduce portion size. In this way, kids can eat satisfying portions while reducing their energy intake.

Health Goals

- Serve a satisfying volume of low-energy-density food.

Suggestions

- Suggestions to reduce portion size are given below:

  a. Serve soup or salad before the main course.
  b. Use small-sized plates (9 in. diameter), bowls (½ to 1 serving size), and glasses (4–8 oz.).
  c. Serve food on individual plates instead of placing serving dishes on the table.
  d. Do not force your child to "clean the plate."

- If your child asks for a second serving, give him or her low-energy-density food such as vegetables or whole-grain food.

- Read "Energy Density" and "Recommended Portion Size" in chapter 10.

Skipping Breakfast

How often does your child skip breakfast?

Knowledge

- About half of schoolchildren aged nine to fifteen reported that they did not eat breakfast on school mornings, preferring to sleep a little later.

- A positive relationship exists between the frequency of skipping breakfast and weight status. Children and adolescents who skipped breakfast were heavier than those who ate breakfast regularly. This was true not only in overweight children but also in children who were not overweight (Berkey et al. 2003, 1258–1266).

- Studies have shown that eating breakfast improves a child's concentration level at school (Hoyland et al. 2009, 220–243).

- Some overweight individuals try to lose weight by skipping breakfast, but this does not work. People who are trying to lose weight are more successful if they have a regular breakfast. The reasons may include the following:

  a. Skipping breakfast may slow down the body's metabolic rate ("starvation mode").
  b. The children are more likely to snack, and the snacks are more likely to be energy heavy.
  c. They may end up overeating at lunchtime.

- A recent study from Great Britain reported that 26 percent of children who skipped breakfast regularly were at a higher risk of developing type 2 diabetes. They had slightly higher blood sugar levels and were more likely to be insulin resistant than those who ate breakfast regularly (Donin et al. 2014).

Health Goal

- Do not skip breakfast or lunch. Eat three meals a day.

Suggestions

- Have children wake up a little earlier and eat a healthy breakfast every day.
- Whole-grain cereals, oatmeal, or whole-wheat toast, topped with fruits and vegetables, along with low-fat milk, are good choices for breakfast.

Eating and Watching TV

Does your child eat while watching TV?

Knowledge

- Research shows that overweight children are more likely than normal-weight children to eat in front of the TV (Robinson 1999, 1561–1567).
- Watching TV while eating may contribute to obesity for the following reasons:

  a. Children who watch TV while eating tend to overeat, because they may be unaware of how much they have eaten. A research study showed that on average, eating while distracted increased the amount eaten by about 10 percent. It also increased the amount a person ate at a later meal by more than 25 percent (Wiecha et al. 2006, 436–442).
  b. TV food commercials may encourage viewers to eat more.
  c. Research suggests that TV watching may reduce the resting metabolic rate in both obese and nonobese children (Dietz et al. 1994, 556–559).

Health Goal

- Do not eat while watching TV.

Suggestions

- Make a "no TV" rule during meals (or snacking).
- Remove TVs from the dining room, as recommended by the AAP.

Bedtime Snacks

How often does your child eat bedtime snacks?

Knowledge
- Complete digestion of food takes three to four hours. Routine unhealthy bedtime snacks can be dangerous in the weight-loss effort, because there is no time to burn extra calories taken in prior to sleep (a low-energy activity state).
- Some children want a bedtime snack as a stall tactic.
- Although regular bedtime snacks should not be served, if the child is genuinely hungry, occasional healthy snacks can provide better sleep and additional nutrition.

Health Goal
- Do not allow bedtime snacks, especially those that are high in fat or sugar.

Suggestions
- Serve dinner at least three hours before bedtime.
- If your child is hungry at bedtime, serve healthy, low-calorie snacks: whole-grain bread, whole-grain cereal and low-fat milk, air-popped popcorn, frozen yogurt, baked potato chips, graham crackers and low-fat milk, a piece of fruit, or vegetable sticks.
- Do not serve high-calorie snacks like high-fat cheese on crackers, ice cream, regular potato chips, chocolate chip cookies, or sugary cereals.

Nutrition Facts Labels

How often do you read the nutrition facts label on food packages?

Knowledge

- Learning how to check the labels will enable you to buy healthier food for your family.

- As an initial step to reduce calorie intake, learn to consistently check the serving size, the calories, the percent daily value (DV) for fat, and the sugar content (fig. 5.1).

  a. Serving size. The information on the label is based on one serving size. One serving size is not necessarily what you are going to eat. If you think you are going to eat two servings, multiply the numbers given for calories, percent DV (shown as %DV in the food labels) for fat, and sugar by two.

  b. Calories. In general, 40 Calories is considered low, 100 Calories is moderate, and 400 Calories is high for one serving, but consider how many servings you are going to eat.

  c. Percent DV for fat. You do not need to check the total fat in grams. Check the percent DV for fat. Less than 5 percent is low, and more than 20 percent is high.

  d. Sugar. Make sure that you know the daily sugar allowance for a child (50 g for a ten-year-old) versus that for an adolescent (75 g). Any food containing more than 25 g of sugar in one serving is considered a high-sugar food.

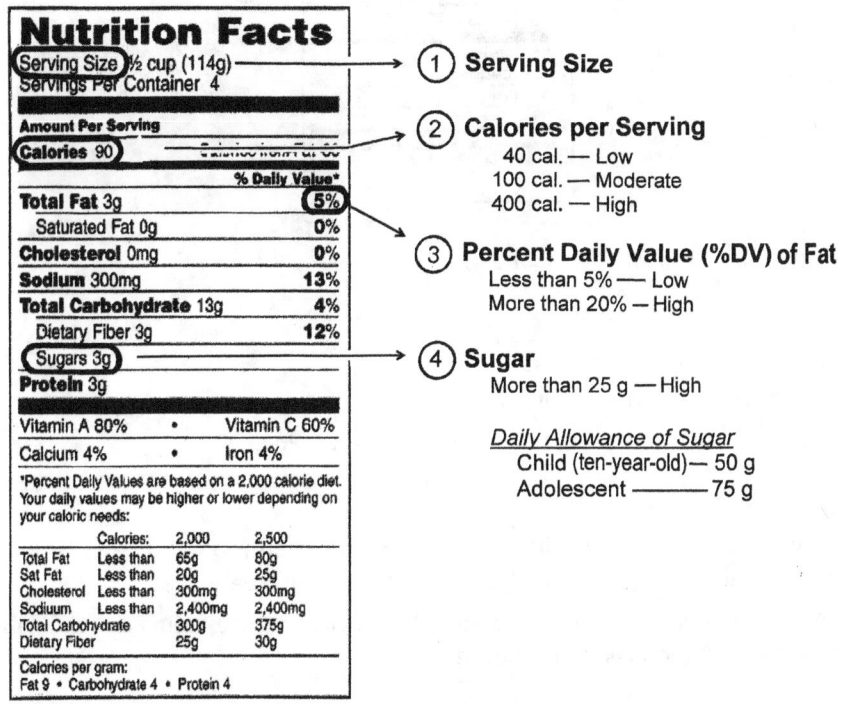

Figure 5.1. Nutrition facts label.

- The Food and Drug Administration (FDA) has proposed a revision of the food label. If adopted, the changes will include the following:

  a. Making the calories and serving size more prominent.
  b. Shifting the position of the %DV to the left of the label.
  c. Information about "added sugars" (many experts recommend consuming fewer calories from added sugar).
  d. Updating the percent DV for sodium, dietary fiber, vitamin D, and potassium.

- When the proposed label is adopted, checking these four elements will be easy, as shown in fig. 5.2.

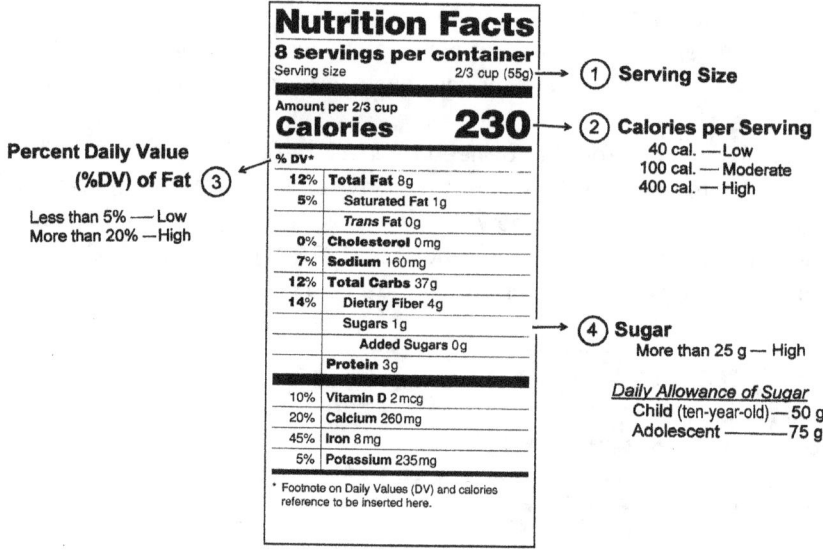

Figure 5.2. Proposed food label.

Health Goals
- Learn how to read the nutrition facts label.
- Always check the nutrition facts label when shopping.

Suggestions
- Ask yourself if you know these four values for each food you serve your children. This will help you develop the habit of checking the label.
- When you feel that you are routinely checking these items on the label, read "Detailed Nutrition Facts" in chapter 10.

Lean Meats

When you buy meat, how often do you look for lean meats?

Knowledge

- Red meats (beef, pork, lamb) are major sources of animal protein, essential amino acids, and vitamins and minerals (such as iron, zinc, vitamins B6 and B12, niacin, riboflavin, selenium, and phosphorus). However, a high concentration of saturated fat in red meat is a health concern. In addition, meat does not provide dietary fiber.
- Health concerns associated with high intake of red meats (and saturated fat) include the following:

  a. An increased risk of heart disease (by raising blood cholesterol levels)
  b. Increased weight problems
  c. Increased risk of cancer (by 20–60 percent)
  d. A higher mortality rate compared to white meat (chicken and turkey) eaters as reported in a recent ten-year study (Sinha et al. 2009, 562–571)

- The USDA grades beef by the percentage of fat content (marbling or fat within muscles) as follows:

  a. USDA Prime is very high in fat (above 8 percent).
  b. USDA Choice is moderately fatty (4–8 percent).
  c. USDA Select is very lean (3–4 percent).

- Most beef offered for sale in supermarkets is US Choice or Select grade. US Prime beef is sold to hotels and upscale restaurants. The fat content of Kobe beef, which refers to cuts of beef from cattle raised in *Kobe*, Japan, and is extremely tender and full flavored, is even higher, at 20–25 percent.
- White meat and fish are excellent sources of protein, but they have much smaller amounts of saturated fat, making them a healthier alternative to red meat.
- Unlike red meat, many fish contain essential fatty acids such as omega-3, which the human body cannot produce. Eating fish may provide some protection from heart disease and stroke.

Health Goal

- Look for lean red meats, or choose poultry or fish instead.

Suggestions

- Look for lean meats, and trim off visible fat before cooking to reduce the amount of saturated fat.
- Reduce consumption of red meat, and eat more poultry (chicken, turkey, pheasant, goose, and duck) and fish.
- Read "Good Fats and Bad Fats" and "Fish and Seafood" in chapter 10.

Frying Food

How often do you deep-fry or pan-fry food when you cook?

Knowledge

- Frying adds calories. Different methods of cooking soak the food in different amounts of fat. Sautéing and stir-frying are healthier methods.

    a. Sautéing uses a small amount of fat in a shallow pan over relatively high heat. It requires constant attention to ensure that the food does not overcook. This method is used to cook small or thinly sliced pieces of vegetables or meat. Only a small amount of fat is absorbed into the food.
    b. Stir-frying uses a minimum amount of fat in a wok at higher temperatures. It requires stirring the food continuously to prevent it from adhering to the surface and burning. Many Chinese dishes are stir-fried.
    c. Pan-frying uses only enough fat to immerse one-third to one-half of each piece of food. This method is used to cook larger pieces of food that are generally breaded or battered. The food is then turned over to cook the other side, so therefore the cooking time is longer. The food soaks up more fat than sautéing or stir-frying.
    d. Deep-frying involves immersing the entire piece of food into a large amount of fat. Using this method, the food soaks up more fat than any other method. Examples of deep-fried food include French fries, fried chicken, onion rings, fried fish, potato chips, donuts, and instant noodles.

- Sautéing and stir-frying are considered healthy ways of cooking, because the food soaks up only a small amount of fat. The nutrients are preserved in the food, because it cooks quickly.
- Deep-frying not only soaks up a lot of fat, but it may produce toxic chemicals, like acrylamide and polycyclic aromatic hydrocarbons, which have been linked to cancer in laboratory animals.

Health Goals

- Do not deep-fry or pan-fry. Use alternative cooking methods.
- Sautéing or stir-frying is the preferred way of cooking with fat.

Suggestions

- Cook food by boiling, steaming, baking, broiling, roasting, or grilling without using fat or oil.
- If you use oil in cooking, stir-fry or sauté the food.
- Read "How to Reduce Fat Intake" in chapter 10.

Low-Fat Products

How often do you choose low-fat or fat-free varieties of food when you shop?

Knowledge

- Many high-fat grocery items come in low-fat versions. By choosing these versions, you can significantly reduce the amount of fat and calories eaten.
- Reduced-fat or fat-free versions are available for many dairy products, including milk, evaporated milk, ice cream, whipping cream, sour cream, cheese, and coffee cream.
- Reduced-calorie products are also available for salad dressings.
- Low-fat versions are not calorie-free or fat-free; some may have only a slightly reduced amount of fat compared to the regular products. Be aware of this, and do not use "low fat" as an excuse to consume large amounts of a reduced-fat food.
- A "fat-free" product should contain less than 0.5 g of fat per serving. Low-fat products should have 3 g of fat or less per serving. If the product is "less fat," it should have 25 (or a greater percentage) percent less fat than the comparison food.

Health Goal

- Look for low-fat or fat-free versions of food products.

Suggestions

- Check the nutrition facts label, even on low-fat versions of food.
- Pay attention to the portion size, and do not overeat low-fat foods.
- Read "How to Reduce Fat Intake" and "Detailed Nutrition Facts" in chapter 10.

Poultry and Fish

How many times a week do you prepare a main dish that contains poultry or fish?

Knowledge

- Poultry and seafood are some of the best sources of protein, because they are usually low in saturated fat. They are much healthier than red meats like beef and pork. Both seafood and poultry can be bought canned, fresh, frozen, or smoked.

- The white meat of poultry is an excellent source of lean protein. Chicken meat is naturally low in sodium. The dark meat is a little higher in fat than white meat, but it contains more iron. The skin of poultry is loaded with saturated fat, though, so remove the skin before cooking. Poultry contains vitamin A, vitamin B complex, and other minerals, although not as many as fish. Good poultry choices include chicken, duck, goose, turkey, partridge, pheasant, and quail.

- Fish is a good source of lean protein, vitamins, and minerals. Fish has many health benefits, primarily owing to its omega-3 fatty acids. Omega-3 fatty acids lower triglyceride levels, lower blood pressure, have an anticlotting effect, and help reduce the likelihood of heart attacks and strokes. Good sources of omega-3 fatty acids are cold-water, oily fish, such as salmon, herring, mackerel, anchovies, and sardines. The American Heart Association (AHA) recommends eating at least two fish meals a week.

Health Goals

- Increase consumption of white meats like poultry and fish.
- Aim to eat fish twice a week.

Suggestions

- The skin of poultry should be removed before cooking, because most poultry fat is found in the skin.
- Use a healthy cooking method to avoid adding fat.
- Avoid large predatory fish such as shark, swordfish, and king mackerel, which are known to contain mercury. Mercury may be dangerous to pregnant women, infants, and children, because it may harm the developing nervous system. Commonly available fish that are low in mercury include shrimp, canned light tuna, salmon, and catfish.
- Read "Fish and Sea Food" in chapter 10.

Eating Restaurant Food

How many times a week does your family eat at a restaurant or eat takeout food (prepared at a restaurant)?

Knowledge

- Eating out has been shown to be an important contributing cause of weight gain. Reducing the frequency of eating out is a proven way to control weight.
- Restaurant food is generally unhealthy because of the following:

  a. It is high in calories due to larger-than-necessary portions and high fat content.
  b. It is usually high in sodium.
  c. People frequently consume a large amount of sugary soft drinks with meals at restaurants, especially at fast-food restaurants where unlimited refills are available.

- Although fast-food restaurants are most frequently cited as places to avoid, many sit-down restaurants prepare foods that are equally poor choices.
- Takeout foods from regular or fast-food restaurants consumed at home have the same consequences.
- You can save a significant amount of money by eating healthier food cooked at home.

Health Goal

- Limit the frequency of eating restaurant food, including takeout food.

Suggestions

- If you have to eat at a fast-food restaurant, consider the following:

  a. Choose a grilled chicken sandwich or a lean roast beef sandwich.
  b. Choose a small or regular portion.
  c. Do not add cheese to your meal.
  d. Use a small amount of salad dressing, or choose a reduced-fat version.
  e. Drink skim or 1 percent milk or water rather than regular soda.

- Read "How to Reduce Fat Intake" in chapter 10.

Family Dinner

How many days in a week does the family eat a home-cooked dinner together?

Knowledge

- Family meals provide multiple benefits in terms of family health, unity, finance, and children's social and academic efforts.
- Home-cooked meals are generally healthier than restaurant food. Several large studies have shown that regular family meals are strongly associated with increased consumption of fruits, vegetables, grains, and other healthy food choices, and they are linked with less consumption of fried or fatty foods and soft drinks (Gillman et al. 2000, 235–240; Neumark-Sztainer et al. 2003, 317–322).
- Family dinners naturally decrease the frequency of eating unhealthy restaurant food and are a proven way to control excess weight. Recent research suggests that family dinners are associated with a reduced risk of childhood obesity (Hammons et al. 2011, e1565–1574).
- Family dinners strengthen the family unit. They offer the opportunity to connect with each other, communicate about family happenings, and give each other time and attention.
- Family meals have an important "protective factor" on children. Parents get to know what their kids are doing, who they are with, and where and when their activities are taking place. These efforts may result in a decreased risk of substance use or delinquency, heightened personal and social well-being, and better academic performance (Sen 2010, 187–196).
- Family dinners save money.

Health Goal

- Have family dinners as often as possible.

Suggestions

- Make sure the TV set is turned off so that everybody participates in the conversation.
- Have fixed mealtimes so that children do not attempt to eat snacks before the meal.

Family Outings

How often do you have family outings on weekends?

Knowledge
- Family outings provide opportunities to be physically active, improve physical fitness, eat healthy food, and build closeness.

Health Goal
- Have fun family outings that include physical activity as often as possible.

Suggestions
- Consider things your family likes to do together that require physical activity. These may include hiking, camping, sports, or community service.
- Try any of the following (modified from the CDC, "Parent brochure: Healthy Kids. Healthy Families," http://www.cdc.gov/HealthyYouth/physicalactivity/brochures/pdf/parent.pdf):

1. A family adventure. See the sights of your community.

    - Try hiking, fishing, canoeing, and berry picking.
    - Try picnicking and camping.
    - Discover the public parks.
    - Visit the zoo.
    - Explore outdoor tourist attractions.

2. Family fitness vacations. Plan an active getaway.

    - Swim at the beach, or bike on a scenic trail.
    - Explore state and national parks.
    - Raft down a river.
    - Take a walking tour of a city.

3. The gift of physical activity. Give a present that encourages activity.

    - Buy a swimsuit or a pair of athletic shoes.
    - Select toys that make kids move, such as a basketball or bicycle.

4. Seasonal celebrations. Welcome each season with fun activities.
    - Winter: Go sledding or build a snowman.
    - Spring: Play whiffle ball or fly a kite.
    - Summer: Run through the sprinkler or jump rope.
    - Fall: Play Frisbee or golf, or hike through a pumpkin patch.

5. Community service. Benefit others while benefiting yourself.

    - Volunteer as a family for your community.
    - Do litter patrol on a nearby road.
    - Help neighbors rake their yard, or team up to clean up a favorite park.

Chapter 6

Setting Goals

Whether it is stopping smoking, stopping drinking, or rehabilitating from drug addiction, most behavioral changes require goal setting, which provides a sense of direction and purpose.

All weight-management efforts start with goal setting. It begins by identifying unhealthy behaviors that need change and working to change them permanently. In weight clinics, clinical staff or counselors will help you set goals for your child. In your case, you set the goals for your child, and you are the substitute for the clinic staff or counselors. You can do as good a job as them, because you will be well educated. The information provided in this book is much more detailed than what you would get from a weight clinic.

Regardless of your child's age, your child cannot or will not change her habits voluntarily or willingly. This is where you come in. Goal setting, in combination with self-monitoring and family support, has proven to be effective for managing a weight problem.

Identifying an Unhealthy Lifestyle

In structured weight-management programs, healthcare providers help families identify a few targeted goals in the areas of nutrition and physical activity. You went through this process and pinpointed the unhealthy behaviors of your child when you answered the lifestyle questions in chapter 3.

Unhealthy lifestyle behaviors can be divided int two groups (table 6.1).
- Group 1: These are unhealthy behaviors that may have contributed to your child's weight problem, and he or she will have to make major changes to these behaviors.
- Group 2: These are unhealthy behaviors of the parents that may have contributed to their child's weight problem. Parents can change these unhealthy behaviors with only minor effort from the child.

The distinction between the two is not always clear-cut. Parents are probably responsible for many of their child's unhealthy behaviors, which likely resulted from lack of parental knowledge or action. All of the unhealthy behaviors listed in table 6.1 contribute to childhood obesity, according to the report of the Expert Committee on Childhood Obesity (Barlow et al. 2007., S164–S192).

Table 6.1 Two categories of unhealthy behaviors contributing to obesity

GROUP 1 Child's contribution	GROUP 2 Parents' contribution

• Insufficient physical activity (less than one hour of moderate activity daily)
• Too much television watching or other screen time (more than two hours a day)
• Consuming too many sugar-sweetened beverages (sodas, fruit drinks, and fruit juices)
• Insufficient consumption of fruits and vegetables (fewer than five servings a day)
• Consuming excessive amounts of fast food, fried food, and chips
• Too many high-fat and high-sugar snacks
• Consuming regular dairy products like cheese
• Unhealthy food choices:
    ○ Drinking whole milk
    ○ Eating white breads or sugary cereals for breakfast
• Unhealthy eating behaviors:
    ○ Skipping breakfast
    ○ Eating while watching television
    ○ Eating bedtime snacks
    ○ Eating large-portion sizes
	• Not buying and serving enough fruits, vegetables, and grain products as main courses and snacks
	• Buying high-sugar drinks (sodas, fruit drinks) and snacks (ice cream, cake, cookies, etc.)
	• Buying high-fat food and snacks (fried food, fast food, chips, etc.)
	• Not buying and serving low-fat versions of dairy products such as milk and cheese
	• Not buying lean meats, poultry, or fish
	• Deep frying or pan-frying when cooking
	• Serving too many potato products
	• Not checking the nutritional facts food label during grocery shopping
	• Frequently eating out or eating "take-out" restaurant food (instead of home-cooked food)
	• Not planning family outings for fun and physical activity
	• Not being a role model for your children

When the unhealthy behaviors are identified, you need to set goals for new habits. The goals should be specific, measurable, realistic, and not painful. Productive and successful goal setting takes thinking and planning, so let us walk through the steps.

Goal Setting for the Child

In setting goals, consider your child's understanding of the weight problem, level of motivation, and the sustainability of the goals.

• Start by ascertaining whether your child understands that he is overweight and how much overweight he is. Discuss why maintaining the current weight is unhealthy and why positive steps need to be taken to improve his weight problem. Encourage your child to express his opinion about the suggestions and how fast he wants to change them.

- Start with small goals. Work on goals that your child is less likely to object to. Unrealistic or overly ambitious goals are likely to fail, thereby jeopardizing the chances of progress.
- Your child may want to take on one or two goals and progress slowly in steps, or she may want to proceed rapidly and change several things at once. Either approach is all right. Respect your child's opinion, and do not force your child to take on bigger goals.
- Proposals for lifestyle changes may be more easily acceptable for preadolescent children than adolescents. You need to handle adolescents differently, because they like to be more independent and have their own ideas. Suggestions for dealing with adolescents are offered in chapter 8.
- Realize that the proposed changes are not just for your overweight child. They will affect all members of the family. Choose behaviors that you are prepared to change and maintain with your child so that you can serve as a role model.
- Be prepared to answer questions your child may have regarding the changes you propose. You may want to review the information in chapter 5.

Healthy Lifestyle Goals for Your Child

Healthy lifestyle goals are listed below. Choose a limited number of goals, and keep in mind that the first five goals are important. The first four constitute the 5-2-1-0 message, and the fifth is a moderation of the SoFAS message. Any goal setting should include attempts to make small changes in all or most of these items.

- Physical activity. Increase the duration of physical activity to an hour or more a day. Give your child options that you can afford and think are safe to do in your neighborhood. He may want to start with thirty minutes and increase the duration gradually.
- Screen time. Reduce the amount of time in front of the TV or computer or playing electronic games to less than two hours per day. Some children have no problem limiting screen time to less than two hours right away, but others may want to reduce the time gradually (for example, from six hours to three or four hours). Either way is all right.
- Sugary drinks. Reduce or eliminate sugary drinks, including soft drinks and fruit drinks. Limit consumption of 100 percent fruit juices. Your child may want to eliminate sodas or other high-sugar drinks completely or reduce the number gradually, depending on how many sweet drinks she has been drinking daily. She may initially want to switch to diet sodas.
- Fruits and vegetables. Aim to eat 5 cups of fruits and vegetables a day. At least 1½ cups of fruit and 2½ cups of vegetables every day are recommended by the AHA and endorsed by the AAP. Increasing consumption of fruits and vegetables is more or less the parents' responsibility; parents should provide them as the main course or as a snack. Start with small steps. Reaching this goal is likely to take longer than the others, so go slow and easy.

- High-fat, high-sugar, and high-salt food. Reduce consumption of these foods and snacks. Take into consideration the number of school lunches that your child purchases, because some school cafeterias serve food similar to that served at fast-food restaurants. Reducing consumption of unhealthy foods will be difficult if they are easily available outside the home. Making lifestyle changes may take time, so go slowly.

- Make healthier choices of milk and bread. Switch whole milk to 1 percent or skim milk. Eat whole-wheat bread and whole-grain cereals for breakfast instead of white bread and sugary cereals.

- Change these behaviors:

  a. Do not skip breakfast.
  b. Do not watch TV while eating.
  c. Do not eat bedtime snacks.
  d. Reduce portion size.

Examples of Initial Goal Setting for the Child

The lifestyle-change forms used in this chapter are from a blank worksheet provided in the appendix (fig. A.3). The form includes the unhealthy behaviors listed by the Expert Committee on Childhood Obesity, and it can be used for any child who needs lifestyle changes. Two examples are presented (fig. 6.1 and 6.2).

Example 1: Johnny

Twelve-year-old Johnny is mildly obese (a BMI slightly above the 95th percentile). He eats breakfast every day, and he eats white bread and drinks whole milk. He watches TV and works on his computer for more than four hours every day after school. He drinks two to three sodas every day. He has no PE class at school, and he does not have regular physical activities at home except for helping his dad in his store occasionally. He loves cheeseburgers and French fries and eats them almost every time they are offered at the school cafeteria. He snacks on chips and crackers while watching TV. He eats at a fast-food restaurant with his family two to three times a week.

Johnny and his parents have agreed to the following goals:

- He will ride his bicycle in the park for at least thirty minutes every day. This will be designated as Goal 1 for self-monitoring purposes (see the next chapter, "Self-Monitoring").
- He will reduce his TV watching and computer time to two hours (Goal 2).
- He will drink water instead of soda (Goal 3).
- He does not want to switch to whole-wheat bread but will try 2 percent milk (Goal 4).
- He will not snack while watching TV (Goal 5).
- He does not want to change school lunch plans at this time, but he will choose a hamburger instead of a cheeseburger (Goal 6).

The goals listed are entered in fig. 6.1. These numbers become convenient in self-monitoring as described in chapter 7. You can add other behaviors to change in the worksheet (like Johnny's Goal 6, which is not listed in the original format).

Name: _____ *Johnny* _____ Date: _____

_1_ Play outside for at least _30_ min every day
    Doing what? _Bicycle ride_ _____

_2_ Reduce TV and other screen time to less than _2_ hours a day
    (Note) _____

_3_ Reduce regular soda or other sugary drinks to _0_ cans/bottles a day
    Will drink ____ diet soda or ____ water
____ Reduce eating hamburgers (or cheeseburgers) to ____ times a week
____ Reduce eating French fries (hash browns, tater tots) to ____ times a week
____ Reduce eating fried foods (fried chicken, fried fish) to ____ times a week
____ Reduce eating chips (___ oz bag) to ___ bags a week (or ____ oz a week)
____ Will eat ____ 1 cup or ____ 2 cups of fruits _____ days a week
____ Will eat ____ 2 cups or ____ 3 cups of vegetables _____ days a week
_4_ Switch whole milk to _2_ % milk or ____ skim milk
____ Will switch to whole-wheat bread
____ Will eat whole-grain cereals for breakfast
____ Will not skip breakfast
_5_ Will not eat while watching TV
____ Will not have after-dinner snacks
_6_ *Hamburger instead of cheeseburger at school cafeteria* _____
____ _____
____ _____
____ _____

Figure 6.1. Goal-setting worksheet for Johnny.

Several unhealthy behaviors are not being addressed right away. Although Johnny wants to eat hamburgers (instead of cheeseburgers) and French fries, his parents have agreed to leave this option the way he wants rather than pressuring him to change. Reducing consumption of hamburgers and fries will become future goals. Johnny is likely to eat chips and crackers, although he will stop snacking on them while watching TV. These habits will also become future targets. Efforts to increase consumption of fruits and vegetables need to be included in the future plan, which requires parents to take the leading role. A plan to reduce the frequency of eating out will be included in the parents' goal setting.

Example 2: Susan

Susan is sixteen years old and extremely obese (a BMI greater than the 99th percentile). She skips breakfast often and watches TV for five to seven hours after school. She seldom exerts herself physically, and she has no friends. She snacks on chips and crackers while watching TV. She says that she is addicted to soda and consumes four to six cans every day. She eats white bread and drinks regular milk. She loves French fries and hamburgers.

Susan and her parents have agreed to the following goals (fig. 6.2):

- She will walk their dog or walk briskly for at least for sixty minutes every day (Goal 1).
- She will reduce her TV time from six hours to four hours (Goal 2).
- She says she cannot stop drinking sodas "cold turkey," so she will reduce them from six to three a day for the time being (Goal 3).
- She will wake up twenty minutes earlier and eat breakfast every day (Goal 4).
- She will not snack when she watches TV (Goal 5).

She will continue to eat white bread and drink whole milk for the time being. She will not agree to reduce eating French fries and hamburgers at this time. She does not like to eat fruits and vegetables, and she does not like whole-wheat bread or reduced-fat milk. These will become her future goals.

```
Name: _____Susan_____ Date: _____

_1_ Play outside for at least _60_ min every day
     Doing what? _Walk dog or walk briskly_____
_2_ Reduce TV and other screen time to less than _4_ hours a day
     (Note) _____
_3_ Reduce regular soda or other sugary drinks to _3_ cans/bottles a day
     Will drink ____ diet soda or ____ water
___ Reduce eating hamburgers (or cheeseburgers) to _____times a week
___ Reduce eating French fries (hash browns, tater tots) to ____times a week
___ Reduce eating fried foods (fried chicken, fried fish) to ____ times a week
___ Reduce eating chips (___oz bag) to ___ bags a week (or ___ oz a week)
___ Will eat ___ 1 cup or ___ 2 cups of fruits _____ days a week
___ Will eat ___ 2 cups or ___ 3 cups of vegetables _____ days a week
___ Switch whole milk to ___% milk or ____ skim milk
___ Will switch to whole-wheat bread
___ Will eat whole-grain cereals for breakfast
_4_ Will not skip breakfast
_5_ Will not eat while watching TV
___ Will not have after-dinner snacks

___ _____
___ _____
___ _____
___ _____
```

Figure 6.2. Goal-setting worksheet for Susan.

As can be seen in these examples, achievable goals may be different from child to child, in part depending on the child's level of motivation. Susan is not as willing to make changes as Johnny is. Her goals are modest initially, but this is an important beginning and better than doing nothing. She still chooses to keep unhealthy behaviors that eventually need to change. Johnny is more motivated and wants to set bigger goals. In goal setting, parents should not pressure their children. It is particularly important not to pressure adolescents who may become rebellious, although the parents can reason with them and convince them to set bigger goals. We discuss dealing with adolescents in chapter 8.

Goal Setting for Parents

Goal setting for parents is as important as setting goals for their obese children. The parents' choices and habits establish and/or contribute to the child's weight problem. It is the parents' responsibility to correct their mistakes and help their child achieve her healthy lifestyle goals. Without parental lifestyle changes, the child will not meet her goals. Parental contributions to their child's weight issues include all the Group 2 behaviors listed in table 6.1.

You can change Group 2 behaviors without much resistance or objection from your child, with strategic grocery store purchases and cooking methods and keeping the home environment healthy. However, certain changes may generate objections from your child, and you may want to discuss the reasons for them in advance. Having your child participate in grocery shopping can be an educational process. Your child may learn how to make healthier choices when involved in choices based on food label evaluation.

Figure A.4 (Parents' Goal-Setting Form) lists most of the unhealthy behaviors that parents can change to help their child to achieve a healthy lifestyle. The form can be used by any family that has an overweight child.

Healthy Goal Setting for Parents

Your goal setting should include changes to correct the behaviors listed under Group 2 in table 6.1. Review them and decide which ones you intend to change. As can be seen in the table, you may have many things to change. The list highlights how you may have contributed to your child's weight problem. The participation of both parents is especially important, because inconsistent messages can significantly reduce the efforts of a committed parent. If one parent cannot be an active participant in the effort, he or she should not block the other parent's efforts.

Johnny's parents set the following goals to help him achieve his own goals:

- They decided to buy only 2 percent milk (Goal 1).
- They will not buy soda and other high-sugar drinks (Goal 2).
- They will remove the TV from Johnny's bedroom (Goal 3).
- They made a new TV rule: no one watches TV more than three hours a day, and parents and children will jointly decide what programs to watch (Goal 4).
- They will limit eating out to once a week (Goal 5).

Figure 6.3 shows how Johnny's parents will change. They still have many other changes to make, but this is a reasonable start.

Date: _____

Grocery Shopping Reminders
___ Check food labels before buying foods
___ Buy more fruit and vegetables
    (Note) _____
_2_ Limit buying sodas
    √ No sodas at all ___ Buy limited number ___ Buy diet sodas only
___ Limit purchase of chips
    ___ No chips ___ Limit number to _____ ___ Buy baked chips only
___ Limit high-sugar/high-fat snacks (ice cream, cakes, cookies, etc)
    Do not buy:_____ Reduce: _____
___ Buy low-sugar varieties of: ___ ice cream, ___ cakes, ___cookies, or _____
___ Buy lean meats and more poultry and fish
    ___ Lean meats ___ More poultry ___ More fish
_1_ Buy more reduced-fat dairy products
    √ Milk, only 2 %, _____ Cheese
___ Limit purchase (and cooking) of potatoes

___ _____
___ _____
___ _____

Food Preparation
___ Make more meal main courses with vegetables
    (Note) _____
___ Make fruits and vegetables available as snacks
___ Do not deep fry or pan-fry foods
___ Reduce serving traditional high-calorie desserts

Home and Family
_3_ Remove TV set from child's bedroom
_4_ Make house TV rule (Describe) *No more than 3 hours of TV at the house*
_5_ Limit eating restaurant foods (including takeout) to _____time(s) a week
___ Have family dinners _____ time(s) a week
___ Have family outings _____ time(s) a month
___ _____

Figure 6.3. Goal-setting worksheet for Johnny's parents.

You will make additional changes for your child and yourself, depending on how well you and your child are doing. This stage will be combined with self-monitoring, which is a vital part of weight-control efforts.

Chapter 7

Self-Monitoring

Setting goals for your child and yourself is the beginning. Unless you monitor your child's behavior on a regular basis, you will not be able to assess whether your child is making progress, and you may find that your child goes right back to where he was when he began. Self-monitoring is the measurement of one's own behavior, and it is the single most important tool in changing any behavior, including rehabilitation from drug addiction or weight management. Children's weight-management programs use the self-monitoring principle in its modified form, and it is fundamentally linked to better outcomes.

For self-monitoring to work, it must be done regularly, accurately, consistently, and honestly. Consistency determines the success or failure. Recent research in obese children reported that high self-monitoring (defined as compliant greater than 50 percent of the time) was associated with a significantly higher weight loss than low self-monitoring (compliant less than 50 percent of the time) over a six-month period. Others have reported similar findings in obese adolescents and obese adults (Germann et al. 2007, 111–121).

In adult weight-loss efforts, a popular monitoring method is writing down everything one eats (a food diary) and everything one does in terms of physical activity (an activity log) and reviewing progress on a regular basis. However, emphasis on this type of detailed food diary or log is impractical in children and adolescents, and it cannot be sustained over a long period. For children, it is better to focus on specific behaviors related to food intake or physical activity and simply record whether certain goals are met on a daily basis. On rare occasions, a detailed food diary and activity log may be justified to determine the cause of the lack of progress (e.g., failing to make progress despite meeting set goals).

In parent-initiated weight-control efforts, self-monitoring has three components:

- Monitoring your child's behaviors. This is the most important task, and it should take place daily. It should be enforced through daily interaction with your child.
- Monitoring your responsibilities in helping your child. This can be done once or twice a week.
- Monitoring your behaviors to improve your own health. This can occur weekly.

Follow Up on Your Child's Progress

As the main supporter of your child's weight-loss efforts, assess whether your child's goals are being achieved. These assessments should take place as frequently as possible to assure you that your child becomes an effective self-monitor. A simple yes or no answer from your child is used, an approach that is expected to be practical and effective. Even then, you need to supervise and encourage your child to sustain the consistency of monitoring. The supervision may take the form of child-parent interaction, and it should take place daily. Younger children will need their parents' assistance in filling out the monitoring calendar, and older children and adolescents require daily interaction with their parents to ensure progress.

In this book, a goal calendar for self-monitoring is used. The calendar has been modified from the work of Drs. Kirk and Bolling of Cincinnati Children's Hospital. A blank version of the form is provided in the appendix (fig. A.5); if you have more than six goals, you can use fig. A.6. A circle may be used for the goals that were fully accomplished and a triangle for the goals that were partially accomplished. Goals that were not achieved can be left blank. Increasing numbers of circles each day or the continued presence of abundant circles are signs of progress.

At the time of the child-parent interaction, check on how well your child is filling out the calendar. This is an occasion to praise your child's good behaviors and communicate with him or her. You can also talk about how the day went for your child. Your responsibilities as a supervising parent are much bigger than your child's in ensuring successful management of his or her weight problem. The high frequency of interaction and your acting as counselors are advantages of parent-initiated weight-control efforts. These may result in better success rates than those seen in professional weight-management clinics.

Figure 7.1 illustrates what the self-monitoring calendar for Johnny may look like. As you recall, Johnny set six goals, and these are shown at the bottom of the calendar with numbers assigned to them (fig. 7.1). If Johnny rode his bicycle for thirty minutes on a particular day, he would circle number 1. If he did not spend more than two hours watching TV or doing computer work, he would circle number 2, and so on. If he had a soda on a particular day, he would leave number 3 blank. If he had a child-parent interaction that day, "CP" would be circled. As indicated by the circles in fig. 7.1, Johnny is fulfilling most of his goals on most of the days, and his new lifestyle has been sustained for a week. Not surprisingly, such compliance is associated with regular child-parent interaction.

SUN	MON	TUE	WED	THU	FRI	SAT
(1)(2)(3) (4)(5) 6 (CP)	(1) 2 (3) (4) △5 (6) (CP)	(1)(2)(3) (4)(5)(6) (CP)	1 (2)(3) (4)(5) 6 (CP)	(1)(2)(3) (4)(5)(6) CP	△1 △2 (3) (4)(5)(6) (CP)	(1)(2)(3) (4)(5) 6 (CP)
(1)(2)(3) (4)(5) 6 CP	(1) △2 (3) (4) 5 (6) (CP)	(1)(2)(3) (4)(5)(6) (CP)	(1) △2 3 (4)(5)(6) (CP)	1 2 3 4 5 6 CP	1 2 3 4 5 6 CP	1 2 3 4 5 6 CP
1 2 3 4 5 6 CP	1 2 3 4 5 6 CP	1 2 3 4 5 6 CP	1 2 3 4 5 6 CP	1 2 3 4 5 6 CP	1 2 3 4 5 6 CP	1 2 3 4 5 6 CP
1 2 3 4 5 6 CP	1 2 3 4 5 6 CP	1 2 3 4 5 6 CP	1 2 3 4 5 6 CP	1 2 3 4 5 6 CP	1 2 3 4 5 6 CP	1 2 3 4 5 6 CP
1 2 3 4 5 6 CP	1 2 3 4 5 6 CP	1 2 3 4 5 6 CP	1 2 3 4 5 6 CP	1 2 3 4 5 6 CP	1 2 3 4 5 6 CP	1 2 3 4 5 6 CP

Use a circle for fully accomplished goal and a triangle for partially accomplished goal.

CP = Child-Parent Interaction

Goal Code
1 = Bicycle ride for 30 minutes
2 = Television and computer to < 2 hr
3 = No more sodas
4 = Switch to 2% milk
5 = No snacking while watching TV
6 = Hamburger instead of cheeseburger

Figure 7.1. Johnny's self-monitoring calendar. Modified from S. Kirk and C. Bolling, "Practical Strategies in a Clinical Setting for Promoting Lifestyle Changes in Overweight Youth." *Obesity Management* 3, no. 6 (2007): 272–282.

Tips for Successful Self-Monitoring

- Parents should supervise the child until he or she learns how to fill in the self-monitoring calendar. The extent of supervision will vary with the age of the child. Younger children require complete supervision, preadolescent children require assistance initially before they become accustomed to the practice, and adolescents prefer doing it without the parent's help.

- Self-monitoring has to be done every day for maximum effect. Every day, examine how your child did that day. You and your child can talk about what she did that day and go over whether her behavior has been consistent with the goals. The child-parent interaction can be established as a monitoring goal, as in Johnny's case (fig. 7.1).

- It is important to remember that the interaction between you and your child should be stress-free. Do not criticize your child for not having accomplished every goal. Be patient, and encourage and praise your child for what he has accomplished. When your child starts to look forward to your daily interactions to show off his accomplishments, it is a strong sign of progress.

- Use this occasion to get to know other aspects of your child's life. This will help maintain an open line of communication with your child and may strengthen bonds among your family members.

- When initial goals are routinely met and healthy behaviors become routine, families may add or modify goals to make further progress. If there are circles around most of the numbers for a month or two, your child may proceed with additional goal setting.

- Once major unhealthy behaviors have been corrected, you should see improvement in the weight status of your child. It may not be weight loss. Even maintaining current weight or achieving a lower rate of weight gain is a sign of progress.

- It will take a variable amount of time to correct an unhealthy habit. If your child has many unhealthy behaviors, you may need to reset goals several times, because your child may not be able to incorporate a particular change into her daily routine.

Adjusting Your Child's Goals

You may need to adjust your child's goals when either he or she successfully achieves goals or, alternatively, does not show any improvement in his or her weight status.

- For example, if your child initially decides to reduce screen time from six hours to four and meets that goal without any problems, you may want him or her to reduce screen time to two or three hours.

- If your obese child starts walking for thirty minutes a day and is doing it consistently, you may want to increase the time to forty-five or sixty minutes or increase the intensity.

- If your child appears to be adhering to the 5-2-1-0 message and his or her weight status is not changing, consider increasing the physical activity to ninety minutes or even two hours per day and/or reducing screen time to less than two hours.

Follow-up on Johnny's Case

Four weeks later, Johnny shows no change in his weight. He continues to ride his bicycle, he has stopped drinking soda, and he limits his TV time to two hours. He drinks 2 percent milk without complaint. When he initially set his goals, he was frequently eating fast food and chips. Clearly, the time has come for Johnny to make more changes. He will continue with his TV time goal of two hours, continue to avoid soda, drink 2 percent milk, and eat breakfast each morning. He and his mother agree to modify his goals as follows (fig. 7.2):

- He will increase his bike riding to an hour (new Goal 1).
- He will keep his TV watching and computer work at two hours (remains as Goal 2).
- He will continue to not drink sodas (remains as Goal 3).
- He will switch to whole-wheat bread (new Goal 4).
- He will continue not eating while watching TV (remains as Goal 5)
- He will further limit eating hamburgers and French fries to two times a week (new Goals 6 and 7).
- He will not eat chips at all (new Goal 8).
- He will eat more fruits and vegetables (with his parents providing them) (new Goals 9 and 10).

Name: _____Johnny_____ Date: _____

_1_ Play outside for at least _60_ min every day
    Doing what? __Bike ride_____

_2_ Reduce TV and other screen time to less than _2_ hours a day
    (Note) _____

_3_ Reduce regular soda or other sugary drinks to _0_ cans/bottles a day
    Will drink _____ diet soda or _____ water

_6_ Reduce eating hamburgers (or cheeseburgers) to _2_ times a week

_7_ Reduce eating French fries (hash browns, tater tots) to _2_ times a week

___ Reduce eating fried foods (fried chicken, fried fish) to _____ times a week

_8_ Reduce eating chips (___oz bag) to _0_ bags a week (or _____ oz a week)

_9_ Will eat _√_ 1 cup or ___ 2 cups of fruits _3_ days a week

_10_ Will eat _√_ 2 cups or ___ 3 cups of vegetables _3_ days a week

___ Switch whole milk to ___% milk or _____ skim milk

_4_ Will switch to whole-wheat bread

___ Will eat whole-grain cereals for breakfast

___ Will not skip breakfast

_5_ Will not eat while watching TV

___ Will not have after-dinner snacks

___ _____
___ _____
___ _____

Figure 7.2. Example of goal adjusting for Johnny.

In his case, his earlier goals remain, because the new healthy habits may not have become routine yet. But he added new goals: an increase in bike riding, not eating chips, and eating more fruits and vegetables. He has more goals to monitor. Because everybody in the family is drinking 2 percent milk without complaint, his previous Goal 4 does not have to be relisted.

When your child adjusts and sets new goals, use a new monitoring calendar. Enter the new goals in the bottom part of the calendar. Johnny now has ten goals to monitor. In this case, use the calendar in fig. A.6 instead of fig. A.5.

Follow-Up on Susan's Case

Although Susan is keeping up with her goals, her weight status has not changed in four weeks. There are a number of obvious targets that need to be changed, because many unhealthy behaviors were left when the initial goals were set. Despite the lack of a significant change in her weight, other gains have been made. Her mother regularly joins her for walking. Susan seems to enjoy her mother's company, and they have become closer and are communicating better. Susan and her mother agree to the following goals (fig. 7.3):

Name: _____*Susan*_____ Date: _____

_1_ Play outside for at least _60_ min every day
    Doing what? ___*Walk briskly with mother*_____

_2_ Reduce TV and other screen time to less than _3_ hours a day
    (Note) _____

_3_ Reduce regular soda or other sugary drinks to _0_ cans/bottles a day
    Will drink _1 can_ diet soda or ____ water

_6_ Reduce eating hamburgers (or cheeseburgers) to _2_ times a week

_7_ Reduce eating French fries (hash browns, tater tots) to _2_ times a week

___ Reduce eating fried foods (fried chicken, fried fish) to ____ times a week

___ Reduce eating chips (___oz bag) to ___ bags a week (or ____ oz a week)

___ Will eat ___ 1 cup or ___ 2 cups of fruits _____ days a week

___ Will eat ___ 2 cups or ___ 3 cups of vegetables _____ days a week

_8_ Switch whole milk to _2_% milk or ____ skim milk

_9_ Will switch to whole-wheat bread

___ Will eat whole-grain cereals for breakfast

_4_ Will not skip breakfast

_5_ Will not eat while watching TV

___ Will not have after-dinner snacks

___ _____
___ _____
___ _____
___ _____

Figure 7.3. Example of goal adjusting for Susan.

- She will walk with her mother for sixty minutes at a faster pace (new Goal 1).
- She will further reduce her TV time to three hours a day (new Goal 2).
- She will stop drinking regular soda and switch to one can a day of diet soda (new Goal 3).
- She will not skip breakfast (remains as Goal 4).
- She will continue to not snack when she watches TV (original Goal 5).
- She will limit eating hamburgers and French fries to twice a week (new Goals 6 and 7).
- She will switch to 2 percent milk (new Goal 8) and whole-wheat bread (new Goal 9).

While Susan has shown some motivation by adding new goals, she will retain her old goals and work on them. She has not included increasing consumption of fruits and vegetables, so these will become future goals. Susan will have to use a new monitoring calendar (fig. A.6) to monitor her nine goals.

Parental Involvement and Self-Monitoring

If your child is not closely supervised, no amount of counseling or goal setting will successfully control her weight. Greater parental commitment will result in more consistent self-monitoring, greater changes in her behaviors, and better chances of succeeding in weight control. This is your opportunity to correct what you failed to do in the past.

As mentioned earlier, there are three ways that you should be involved:
- Daily child-parent interaction to monitor your child's consistency in achieving set goals
- Monitoring your own goals in helping your child achieve his goals
- Self-monitoring your unhealthy behaviors

Daily Child-Parent Interaction

Effective and regular child-parent interaction is the key in weight management. It should occur daily or as often as possible. This is like visiting a weight-management clinic every day, and it explains in part the high success rate in parent-initiated weight-management efforts. As mentioned earlier, it should be a happy, stress-free occasion.

Self-Monitoring to Help Improve Your Child's Behavior

In chapter 6, we discussed parental goal setting as a way to establish a home environment that supports your child's weight-loss goals. These goals are meant to make the child's behavior change easier.

As shown in fig. 6.3, Johnny's parents set the following goals: buying more reduced-fat dairy products, not buying sodas, removing the TV set from Johnny's bedroom, limiting TV viewing to three hours a day, and limiting eating out to once a week.

Parents need to monitor if they are keeping up with their own goals on a regular basis, perhaps weekly. Parents can use the same self-monitoring calendar as the child (fig. A.5) and write their goals in the lower part of the calendar. They should adjust their goals once in a while using fig. A.4. Johnny's parents may want to add the following (not shown in the figure):

- Learn how to read food labels (as Goal 6)
- Buy more fruits and vegetables (as Goal 7)
- Limit high-sugar and high-fat snacks (as Goal 8)

Parent's Self-Monitoring of Unhealthy Behaviors

One highly relevant form of involvement for parents is monitoring their own unhealthy behaviors. Even nonobese parents may have unhealthy lifestyles, thereby setting a poor example for their child. Researchers have shown that the children of self-monitoring parents self-monitor more, and they lose significantly more weight when compared to children whose parents do not self-monitor (Germann et al. 2007, 111–121).

Examples of a Detailed Food Record and Activity Log

Although the simplified method described in this book will work for most families, it may become necessary to make more detailed records of food intake and physical activity, particularly when weight management is not progressing or there is a setback.

Food Record

The most common type of self-monitoring in weight-loss programs is a food record. You write down everything you eat or drink throughout the day. In some adult weight-loss programs, you enter other information, such as eating time, calories consumed, triggers to eating, mood or stress level, and psychological variables relating to the situation. Asking for such additional information is not practical in the pediatric population; it is almost impossible for adults to keep highly detailed daily food records over the long term. For this reason, it is common to ask people to keep a detailed record for a few days each week. An example of a three-day record for a twelve-year-old child is shown in table 7.1.

Table 7.1 Example of a three-day food record for a twelve-year-old boy

DATE	MEAL	FOOD EATEN	HOW MUCH
March 3	Breakfast	Cereal with milk	1 small bowl
		Banana	1 medium
	School lunch	Cheeseburger and French fries	1 each
		Chocolate milk	8 oz
		Pear	1 medium
	Snack	Bag of popcorn (individual)	1
		Popsicles	2
	Dinner	Burritos with ground beef, beans, and cheese	2
		Half-liter Coke	1
		Hard-shell tacos (w/meat)	2
		Potatoes, baked	1 large
		1 piece honeydew melon	1
March 4	Breakfast	Egg (scrambled)	1
		Hash browns (fried)	1
		Sausage links	2
	School lunch	Soft tacos with chicken and cheese	2
		Chocolate milk	8 oz
	Snack	Sundae	1
		Bag of popcorn (individual)	1
		1 fruit punch	1 glass
	Dinner	Chuck steak, broiled	8 oz
		Salad with tomatoes, lettuce, & apple	1 serving
		Macaroni & cheese	1 serving
		Fruit punch	16 oz.
March 5	Breakfast	Bacon	2 slices
		Egg, scrambled	1
		Toast, white bread	3
	School lunch	Turkey sandwich	1
		Chips	1 small bag
	Snack	Coke	1 can
		Cocoa cereal	1 bowl
	Dinner	Spaghetti	2 bowls
		Garlic bread	3 slices
		Milk	1 glass
		Ice cream	1 small bowel

Comments on the Food Record

A professional weight-clinic counselor or a dietitian might have made the following comments about the food record:

1. Overall, the child is not eating enough fruits and vegetables as a main dish or a snack.
2. He is not consuming enough grain products. His food diary indicates that he is far from the goals established by MyPlate.
3. There are too many calories from fatty and sugary food.

Activity Log

Monitoring activity is as important as monitoring food intake, and it is simpler to complete. This includes recording the number of minutes of exercise and the intensity and the duration of sedentary activities like watching TV, playing electronic games, or working on a computer. Some adult weight-loss programs ask participants to write down their emotional or social circumstances each day, such as feeling too depressed to engage in activity, or exercise "buddies" being unavailable that day. An example of a twelve-year-old boy's activity log is presented in table 7.2. "Moderate" describes the activities that make one breathe hard and sweat. Activities that are less intense are "mild," and activities that are more intense are "heavy."

An important development that helps individuals monitor their physical activity is the pedometer, which can provide objective data on the number of steps taken daily. For most children, twelve thousand steps may be adequate.

Table 7.2 Example of activity and screen time record

DATE	TIME (DURATION)	TYPE OF ACTIVITY	INTENSITY	WITH WHOM
July 14	10:00–11:00 a.m.(60 min.)	PE class	Moderate	
	4:00–4:30 p.m. (30 min.)	Bicycle riding	Moderate	Tom, Ellen
	6:00–9:00 p.m. (3 hr.)	TV watching		Alone
July 15	4:00–5:20 p.m. (80 min.)	TV game		Alone
	7:00–9:00 p.m. (2 hr.)	TV watching		Tom
July 16	4:00–6:00 p.m. (2 hr.)	Played outside	Mild	Friends
	7:00–8:30 a.m.(90 min.)	Electronic game		Friends
	8:30–9:00 p.m. (30 min.)	Walked dog	Mild	Alone

Comments on the Activity Log

A weight-clinic counselor may have made the following comments:

1. This child has spent too much time in sedentary activities such as watching TV and electronic games.
2. He did not have enough exercise, especially on July 15. He needs to increase physical activity to at least one hour of moderate-intensity activity (longer if the activity is less than moderate).

CASE 3

AJ, a 9-year-old boy, was referred to the Weight Management Clinic for mild obesity. His BMI was 23.0, a little above the 95th percentile. He also had noticeable acanthosis nigricans, which was first detected by a school nurse. There was a family history of diabetes on both sides of the family. His mother is single and works full time. AJ lives with his mother in an apartment building.

Lifestyle questionnaires showed that AJ watches TV from the time he comes home from school until the time his mother comes home from work around 6 PM. After dinner he continues to watch TV with his mother for another hour or two before he goes to bed. Although there are many children his age in the housing project, he does not like to play with them. AJ and his mother almost never go to fast food restaurants. AJ likes to drink sodas and fruit drinks and his mother consistently stocks enough for him to drink when he is home alone. He eats different types of cereal for breakfast every day and his lunches are from the school cafeteria. The family eats white bread and drinks whole milk.

In a short educational session, AJ and his mother learned that they were practicing unhealthy habits at home. The main problem is the lack of physical activity (inactivity) due to too many hours of TV watching, and this problem is compounded by consuming too many sugary drinks. They also learned that one can of soda contain about 150 Calories and that AJ needs to exercise for at least an hour to burn these calories in order to prevent him from gaining weight.

Two lifestyle goals were settled upon: (1) to reduce TV watching and (2) to reduce the consumption of soda. They also decided to switch to 1 % milk.

Within a month, AJ lost about 4 pounds. This brought his BMI to slightly below the 95th percentile. When seen 2 months later after having spent a month with his father who lives in a different city, AJ had gained more than 10 lb. of weight and his BMI returned to its original level prior to starting his weight loss management strategy.

This case illustrates one frequent barrier to weight control efforts—when children are not given consistent messages from all the adults who supervise them (e.g. when grandparents baby sit after school or when a child spends weekends or summer months with a separated parent)—many of the newly acquired healthy lifestyles are lost over time. It is important to recognize potential barriers or spoilers in your child's weight management efforts and make an effort to avoid such barriers. It is important for parents to ask all of the child's care givers to follow similar guidelines as those in the primary home in order to maintain newly acquired healthy lifestyles.

Chapter 8

As the Journey Continues

The effort to control weight in an overweight or obese child is a long process. It may be weeks or months before you see any evidence that your efforts are paying off. Regardless of how quickly or slowly you achieve success, it is critical that your efforts not be derailed and that you stay the course. We consider the situations that you may face in the process and offer information that will help you persevere through difficult times.

Signs of Succeeding in Weight Control

How do you know if your child is headed in the right direction? If you see a weight reduction in a month or two, your child is doing well. However, frequently, children will not experience any weight loss. You should be satisfied if there is no weight gain. While your child's weight remains steady, his expected natural growth in height may move the BMI toward normal.

In encouraging your child, do not emphasize the weight itself. Emphasize the healthy behavioral changes and achieving the goals you set together. Understandably, you would like to see your child lose weight, because it is a sure sign of positive results, but avoid emphasizing the weight itself. Your child will not lose weight every time you check it. On some days, there may be a slight increase, depending on the accuracy of the scale you are using and when the weight is measured (with respect to meals and restroom activities). This is the natural course of weight-management efforts. If you focus on a number, your child may become discouraged when the number is not seen and may not want to continue the effort. Do not check your child's weight frequently. Assess it once or twice a month on a reliable scale.

Even though the significance of a single measurement of weight is not that important, you can follow your child's collective weight measurements in the course of the weight-control process. Try to control variables in weight measurement as much as possible for meaningful comparison of the serial measurements. You need a reliable scale to start with, and you should use the same scale each time. There are variations even with the same brand. A digital scale is better than a spring-loaded one. Place the scale on a floor that is level and not carpeted. Have your child take off her shoes and remove heavy clothing before stepping on the scale. She should stand in the center of the scale. It is recommended that the measurement be made at about the same time of day, preferably in the morning, before a meal and after a restroom visit. Record the result to the nearest quarter pound and the date. Beware that digital scales may be temperature sensitive; they may show a higher weight in cold temperatures, for example.

Home measurement of height is less reliable than weight measurement, and calculating BMI using home measurements of weight and height is unreliable and unrealistic. When your child visits a doctor, it would be a good time to have her BMI calculated using the doctor's measurements of weight and height.

Encouragement is the key to the success. Praise your child for any progress he or she has made. Even if you do not see a reduction in weight, any improvement in any behaviors that are risk factors is a positive sign and deserving of praise. Look for something positive, and encourage your child to maintain her efforts. Box A.1 in the appendix lists one hundred ways to praise a child.

The following are considered signs of positive weight-management results:

- Mastering and maintaining newly acquired healthy behaviors (even in the absence of noticeable weight change)
- Weight maintenance; no weight gain
- Small weight loss
- Improved risk factors, such as increased HDL cholesterol, decreased LDL cholesterol, decreased triglyceride level, reduced blood pressure, and so on

It is strongly recommended to have your child's doctor check risk factors such as blood sugar, cholesterol, triglycerides, and blood pressure before starting a weight-loss effort and recheck them in three to six months. Many overweight children and their parents are more concerned with elevated cholesterol levels or high blood pressure than being overweight, because they have heard so much about the health effects. The results of these risk factors will show you the true risks of your child's health and give you an additional tool in managing his weight. For example, if any risk factor is abnormal, use this to motivate your child to change his behavior. When the risk factor improves, use this to praise your child.

Weight-Loss Goals

What should your child's target weight be, and how fast should he get there? The target weight of any weight-control effort is to reach the BMI of the 85th percentile or less. It is important not to aim to reach the weight goal quickly. Take the time to reach the target gradually; three to six months may be ideal for a mildly obese child. It may take longer for a moderately obese child to reach the target. For overweight and mildly obese children, the Expert Committee on Childhood Obesity recommends maintaining the current weight as the goal; it will reduce the child's BMI as she grows. For severely obese children, gradual weight loss is ideal. Don't be too ambitious or aggressive with weight loss, and remember that the weight-control effort is a long process. Be satisfied with no major weight gain; it is a positive sign of your efforts.

Large weight losses should not be aimed for or expected in weight-control efforts at home. Attempts to achieve large losses in a short period can result in serious medical complications and should be undertaken only under the close supervision of a pediatrician, family practitioner, or multidisciplinary weight-management clinic staff. If the average weight loss is more than 2 lb. per week in any age group, it should be brought to the attention of a pediatrician. It is likely to be associated with practices that may be risky for the child's health (skipping meals, purging, fasting, excessive exercise, and use of laxatives, diet pills, or weight-loss supplements).

The Expert Committee on Childhood Obesity recommends the following goals for the categories of weight status on different age groups (table 8.1):

- If your child was in the *overweight* (85th to 94th percentile) range when you began your efforts, aim to bring your child's BMI down to less than the 85th percentile. Your child does not need to lose a lot of weight; maintenance of her current weight will likely be sufficient. Small, gradual weight loss while consuming a healthy, adequate-calorie diet is all right.

- If your child was *obese*, the general weight goal for all ages is to reduce weight until the BMI is less than the 85th percentile. However, many clinicians will be satisfied with achieving a BMI between the 85th and 95th percentile (i.e., in the overweight range), although continued efforts to further reduce BMI should be made.

Table 8.1 Target weight according to age and weight status*

AGE	WEIGHT STATUS	TARGET WEIGHT
2—5 yr.	Overweight	Weight maintenance (until BMI < 85th percentile)
	Obese	Weight maintenance (or loss of < 1 lb./mo. while on healthy diet)
	BMI > 21	Gradual weight loss < 1 lb./mo.
6—11 yr.	Overweight	Weight maintenance (until BMI < 85th percentile)
	Obese	Weight maintenance (until BMI < 85th percentile) (or gradual loss ~ 1 lb./mo.)
	Severe obesity	Weight loss less than 2 lb./wk.
12—18 yr.	Overweight	Weight maintenance (until BMI < 85th percentile)
	Obese	Weight loss until BMI < 85th percentile) (or gradual loss less than 2 lb./wk.)
	Severe obesity	Weight loss less than 2 lb./wk.

* From S. E. Barlow and the expert committee, "Expert Committee recommendations regarding the prevention, assessment, and treatment of child and adolescent overweight and obesity: summary report." *Pediatrics* 120 (2007): S164–S192.
Overweight, BMI 85th–94th percentile; obese, BMI ≥ 95th percentile; and severely obese, BMI ≥ 99th percentile.

- If your child's BMI was higher than the 99th percentile (*severe obesity*) or close to it, gradual weight loss is emphasized. In this case, the chances of successful weight control are reduced, in part because often the child cannot be removed from the environment that promoted the obesity in the first place. That said, severely obese children can succeed in controlling their weight if properly supported by their parents and family.

If your child is severely obese, seek medical advice from your child's physician, including referral to a weight-management center. Severely obese children are likely to show signs of metabolic syndrome, and close medical supervision of their weight-loss efforts is generally indicated. Some of these children may be candidates for bariatric surgery. Chapter 11 describes medications and surgeries for severely obese adolescents that can be carried out by tertiary weight-management centers. While these may eventually become options for some children, this should not deter you from starting the weight-loss efforts described here.

Incentives and Rewards

When your child reaches her set goals, offer verbal praise and encouragement. Verbal praise motivates and encourages your child to make lifestyle changes. One hundred different ways to praise your child are presented in the appendix (box A.1).

You may agree to a nonfood incentive or reward for your child when goals are achieved and mastered. Box 8.1 shows a list of age-appropriate incentives and rewards for meeting set goals. For a reward to be effective, it must be age appropriate and something the child wants but does not get to do often. Food should never be used as a reward or punishment. For example, buying your overweight child ice cream or a dessert may give the impression that these foods are more desirable than those you are encouraging him or her to eat.

Setbacks

On any journey, you may encounter detours or get lost along the way. Setbacks are a normal part of any behavioral change, and they are the rule rather than the exception. They should not be viewed as failures. Be prepared to face these challenges with your child before beginning any weight-control program. No matter how hard your child tries to gain control over her food and activity choices, he or she will likely experience some backsliding from time to time. Professor James O. Prochaska of the University of Rhode Island described "relapse" as one of the stages of his well-known "stages of change" (also known as the transtheoretical model, or TTM) that may apply to rehabilitation from drug addiction, alcoholism, smoking cessation, or weight-control efforts. Prochaska's stages of change include (1) precontemplation (not ready), (2) contemplation (getting ready), (3) preparation (ready), (4) action, (5) maintenance, and (6) termination or relapse (Prochaska et al. 1992, 1102–1114). While your goal should be to minimize the number of setbacks, the most important thing is how you handle these situations when they occur.

Box 8.1 Examples of age-appropriate incentives and rewards

YOUNG CHILDREN (Age 5—8)	MIDDLE CHILDHOOD (Ages 8—12)	ADOLESCENTS (Ages 12—19)
Daily stickers	Trip to the park	Buying a music CD or download
"Grab bag" with small, inexpensive items	Planning a day of family activities	Renting or buying a DVD or video download
Playing date with a friend	Time on the telephone or computer	Phone card minutes for a cellphone
Small toy	Going to the movies with friends	Car privileges (for those with a valid driver's license)
Spending nights with friends or relatives	Making a craft with a family member	Taking a break from chores
Staying up late	Sleepover	Going to a concert or other special event with friends
Going someplace alone with a parent or guardian	Taking a break from chores	Materials to decorate bedroom
Special outing (e.g., zoo, amusement park, museum, library, etc.)	Sleeping in a different place in the house	Allowing a special haircut or hairstyle
Arts or craft supplies (e.g., colored chalk, crayons, markers, etc.)	Play a board or card game or doing a puzzle with a family member	Getting nails done or a pedicure
Sleeping in a different place in the house	Go to a sporting event with a family member	Buying a new clothing item
Playing a board or card game or doing a puzzle with a family member	Staying up late	A new magazine subscription
Going skating, swimming, bowling, or playing miniature golf	Buying something special	Going bowling, skating, or to the movies with friends
Going to a park	Going skating, swimming, bowling, or playing miniature golf	Having friends over
	Special outing (e.g., zoo, amusement park or water park, children's museum, etc.)	Extending curfew
	Renting or buying a DVD or video download	Staying overnight at friends' home
	Inviting a friend over to play	Mall trip with friends
		Special outing (amusement or water park
		Extra spending money

Modified from S. Kirk and C. Bolling, "Practical strategies in a clinical setting for promoting lifestyle changes in overweight youth." *Obesity Management* 3, no. 6 (2007): 272–282.

These are the common signs of setbacks in weight-control efforts:

- Noticing a significant weight gain, which would be unexpected based on your monitoring of your child's behaviors
- Behavioral setbacks, such as returning to old habits or sneaking food, which are not as easy to detect as weight gain

How to Manage Setbacks

It is important not to get discouraged or become angry with your child when setbacks occur. Stay calm, and think positively. Even if your child gains a pound or two, this is not a reason to abandon all the progress he or she has made so far. Do not scold your child or blame other family members for these inevitable bumps in the road. Face the challenges by calmly assessing what may have gone wrong and instituting a plan that will help you minimize the risk of repeating it.

You and your child need to think about the source of the problem. Was there an event, a person, or a behavior that contributed to it? Did it happen once, or is it an ongoing issue? Without making a serious effort to identify the cause, you are unlikely to be able to correct it. See if one of the following pertains to your situation:

- Is it the result of minor events that coincidentally occurred in a row? For example, perhaps your child overate at a friend's birthday party and then visited a family gathering where he was not closely monitored. Perhaps your child grabbed unhealthy food in the school cafeteria when he felt stressed about an upcoming exam and did not tell you about it.
- Figure out if the setbacks occur at certain times. For example, do they coincide with Grandma's visits? Did your child visit a grandparent or other relative on a recent weekend or during the holidays?
- Are you stopping by fast-food restaurants and bringing home takeout food because of your busy schedule?
- Have you been on the road during a vacation and had to eat fast food?
- Have you or your child forgotten or neglected your self-monitoring activities in recent days (or weeks)?
- Is your child sneaking junk food when you are not looking? Sneaking food needs to be handled with special care, but it must be addressed and resolved.
- Has your child been inactive due to an illness or injury?
- If the cause is still not clear after considering all of these possibilities, you may want to start a food diary and activity log. Such diligence can help you identify specific problem areas and why they might be happening (see chapter 7).

Refocus your efforts on making lifestyle changes, and help your child rebuild confidence. Even if you have not been successful in pinpointing the cause of the setback, your child should continue his commitment to eating healthy and being physically active.

- Keep monitoring your child's progress in the weeks and months ahead. Strengthen your child-parent interaction, and if you have not been monitoring on a regular basis, start doing it regularly. Make sure that you and your child do not fall back into unhealthy habits.
- Don't let your child give up on the weight-control process. There may be more obstacles that temporarily derail your child, so help him understand that it is a process that takes time. Encourage him and reaffirm his decision to continue with the weight-control program.
- Reassure your child that you are there for her and want to help in any way you can. Revive her motivation by praising what she has accomplished thus far. Cite improvements that she has made with cholesterol levels, blood pressure, blood sugar, blood triglycerides, and so forth.
- Allow your child to help figure out what went wrong, and work together on a plan to prevent it from happening again.
- Let your child help with meal planning, food shopping and preparation, and family activity planning. This will help him learn to make good decisions by following your example.

Enlist the help of others. Even after evaluating the setback, you may not clearly identify its cause. If this is the case, find someone who can help you with the changes you need to make. Your pediatrician, nurse, dietitian, or behavioral psychologist may be able to help.

Sneaking Food

If your child does not make progress in her weight-management efforts despite her apparent attempts, consider the possibility that your child is sneaking food. Your child could be indulging at a friend's home or may be purchasing treats when you are not around. You might notice food disappearing in your house. This is going to sabotage both your child's past and ongoing efforts to control weight.

When sneaking is detected or suspected, it is important that you confront your child calmly. Here are some suggestions on how to approach this conversation:

- Let him know that you want to discuss an important issue in the weight-control effort. You might start by saying, "I have noticed something that worries me. I can't understand why you are gaining weight when you seem to eat so healthy." Tell him that you want to help, not condemn. Do not accuse, become angry, or threaten to punish him.

- Once you have opened the conversation, sit back and listen to what your child has to say. You may hear denial. If so, tell her that you love her and are always there if she wants to talk. It may take some time before your child is ready to open up to you.

- Remind your child that no food is off-limits and that anything is OK in moderation. Let your child know that he should not feel embarrassed about craving certain foods or about overindulging. Explain that sticking with new kinds of healthy food is not easy and that everybody has difficulty eating healthy all the time. Let him know that you will not be angry if he occasionally eats unhealthy food. Tell him that when he faces cravings for a certain food, he should ask for it. You may want to praise him for asking and give him healthy choices among the foods that he wants. The bottom line is to make sure your child knows that you understand what he is going through.

- Point out that her behavior is counterproductive to achieving the weight-loss goals she has set for herself and that it is ruining her past good efforts.

- Find out why he might be sneaking food. Children may sneak food for various reasons:

  a. He may have anxiety over issues with friends.
  b. She may be sad or lonely.
  c. He might have been teased or bullied.

- If the problem persists, consult a health professional. Sneaking food is often a symptom of an underlying emotional issue or depression, so it is important to seek professional help if you cannot resolve the behavior by yourself.

Bullying

Some obese children have to deal with more than just controlling their weight. They may be teased or bullied at school. Bullying is repeated, aggressive behavior engaged in to intentionally hurt another person physically or mentally.

Direct bullying involves physical aggression such as shoving, poking, throwing things, slapping, punching, kicking, beating, pulling hair, and pinching. Indirect bullying (social aggression) is characterized by socially isolating the victim. It may include spreading gossip, refusing to socialize with the victim, bullying other people who wish to socialize with the victim, name-calling, the "silent treatment," false rumors, or laughing at the victim.

How Prevalent is Bullying?

Since it tends to be hidden, the exact prevalence of bullying is not known, though some patterns have come to light. Overweight adolescents are more likely than normal-weight children to be victims of bullying. According to a Canadian study on children eleven to sixteen years old, almost 11 percent of normal-weight children and 19 percent of obese children reported that they were victims of bullying (Janssen et al. 2004, 1187–1194). Obese children are also more likely to be bullies (the perpetrators) of other children. By bullying other kids, they avoid being bullied themselves.

What Are the Effects of Bullying?

The effects of bullying can be wide ranging, long lasting, and even fatal. Both victims and bullies experience emotional and social consequences.

- Victims are more likely to do poorly in school, have low self-esteem, be depressed, turn to violent behaviors to protect themselves, or commit vengeful acts on their bullies.
- Kids who bully are more likely to do poorly in school, smoke and drink alcohol, and commit crimes in the future.
- Bullying can cause loneliness, depression, and anxiety. Bullying can keep children from wanting to take part in activities. This is particularly detrimental for obese children, because the only things left for them are food and TV, further explaining why their physical activity levels are low.
- According to the meta-analysis of results from several countries, bullies and victims of school bullying are two times more likely than their uninvolved peers to show negative symptoms such as headache, abdominal pain, dizziness, sleeping problems, poor appetite, bedwetting, vomiting, fatigue, or feeling tense (Gini et al. 2009, 1059–1065).
- Children or adults who are persistently subjected to abusive behavior are at risk of stress-related illnesses that can lead to depression and suicide. Some school shootings are believed to be related to bullying. An investigation undertaken by the US Secret Service found that in more than two-thirds of school shooting cases, the

perpetrators were victims of bullying (US Secret Service and US Department of Education. May 2002).

- Both bullies and victims tend to have difficulty forming adult relationships and suffer an increased risk of depression.

Signs of Bullying and What to Do

Recognizing the signs of bullying is an important step in breaking the chain. Signs include increased stress, depression, unexplained bruising, recurrent abdominal pain, vomiting, frequent or repeated accidents, hyperventilation, submissive behavior, and refusal to attend school.

If you are concerned that your child may be a victim or a perpetrator, seek advice from the school or a doctor/pediatrician. Many schools have antibullying campaigns in place. Studies prove that school-based interventions to reduce bullying are effective (Vreeman al. 2007, 78–88).

What Can Parents Do to Prevent Bullying at School?

Parents can take action to prevent bullying at school, according to the National Crime Prevention Council (National Crime Prevention Council. 2002):

- Teach kids to solve problems without using violence, and praise them when they do.
- Give children positive feedback when they behave well, which builds their self-esteem. Give them the self-confidence to stand up for what they believe in.
- Ask your children about their day, and listen when they talk about school, social events, classmates, and problems they have.
- Take bullying seriously. Many kids are embarrassed to say they have been bullied. You may have only one chance to step in and help.
- If you see bullying, stop it right away, even if your child is the bully.
- Encourage your child to help others who need it.
- Don't bully your children or bully others in front of them. Many times kids who are bullied at home react by bullying other kids. If your children see you hit, ridicule, or gossip about someone, they become more likely to do so themselves.
- Support a bullying prevention program in your child's school. If your school doesn't have one, consider starting one with other parents, teachers, and concerned adults.

Dealing with Adolescent Children

Puberty and adolescence overlap, but they describe different aspects of development:

- Puberty is the process of *physical* changes by which a child's body becomes an adult body capable of reproduction. Puberty usually occurs in girls between the ages of ten and fourteen. In boys, it generally occurs between the ages of twelve and sixteen.
- Adolescence is the period between the beginning of puberty and adulthood. It is a time of *psychological* maturation, during which a person becomes "adult-like" in behavior. Adolescence is roughly the period between thirteen and nineteen. The adolescent experiences physical changes as well as emotional, psychological, social, and mental changes.

Differences between Children and Adolescents

Effective parenting skills differ according to the child's age, especially in weight-control efforts:

- Educating and motivating your preadolescent child is relatively easy, and you are well equipped to deal with that. He or she tends to accept and follow what you tell him or her in order to please you. Preadolescent overweight children are more likely to respond to parental messages and cues and to make efforts to change unhealthy behaviors.
- Adolescents, on the other hand, may be difficult to deal with. This is because of the rapid changes occurring in physical, emotional, psychological, and social aspects of their life. They are physically growing, and they want to be independent and treated with respect. As adolescents struggle to establish their identity independent of parents and other adults, they commonly exhibit resistance to and resentment of authority figures. They look to their peers for approval and reinforcement.

There are differences in the success rates in weight-management efforts in children versus adolescents, primarily related to the issues mentioned above. In general, it is easier to succeed in making lifestyle changes when the effort starts during childhood. Less than 50 percent of obese children and more than 80 percent of obese adolescents become obese adults (Cuo and Chumlea 1999, 145S–148S). This fact reflects the relative difficulty in reversing adolescent obesity and the importance of efforts to manage obesity before children reach adolescence.

Suggestions for Dealing with Adolescents

The parent-centered helping style used for motivational changes in children may no longer work. Your teenager has grown physically and has become independent in thought and behavior. Teenagers do not want to be told what to do. They see this as "nagging" and may become rebellious.

Child psychologists offer the following suggestions for dealing with adolescents:

- When you have a problem, appeal to their sense of reason. Lead them into giving you the right answers, and ask them to consider doing the right thing. At the same time, offer words of optimism, affirmation, and confidence in their ability to make changes. Give them the freedom of choice, and encourage a change based on their decisions as long as it is in the right direction. This approach works better than criticizing and telling them what to do.
- Consciously take opportunities to communicate with them. Communication should involve careful listening without judgment, concession, and compromise rather than promoting your ideas. This gives them the respect they feel they deserve. This approach may work in motivating your overweight adolescent to do the right thing.
- Adolescents do not think about long-term consequences; they are focused on the present. Although you should talk with them about the health consequences of being obese, they may not be convinced. They may be more receptive to discussing issues that are currently bothering them. For example, they may lack stamina in sports and may be getting short of breath before their nonobese peers. They are likely to be preoccupied about their physical appearance. Think about what might be bothering them about being obese, even if they do not admit this to you.

Dealing with Unmotivated and Indifferent Adolescents

Lack of motivation and indifference are common causes of weight-control failure in adolescents, and there are several reasons for it:

- Only 20 percent of obese teens have correctly recognized that they have a weight problem. Enlisting the support of overweight patients who are not concerned about their own weight is not likely to be successful. In such cases, making them realize that they have a weight problem is the first step in the weight-control effort.
- Adolescents may eat more meals outside the home due to their busy schedules, and their parents can no longer monitor what they eat most of the time.
- Adolescents may not have been educated about or exposed to healthy lifestyle habits, and they do not perceive a link between their lifestyle and their weight.
- Many obese adolescents lack family role models for healthy living. One or both parents may be obese, but they are not making efforts to change their lifestyle regardless of what they ask their child to do.

What *Not* to Do

If your obese adolescent cannot be motivated to control his weight, you probably need professional counsel. It is not easy even for trained child psychologists to motivate unmotivated adolescents. For untrained parents, the success rate is much lower, and some parental efforts may even make things worse. Even if you cannot successfully motivate your child, take steps to avoid making the situation worse.

Do not treat your adolescent like you treated him or her five years ago. Treat your child with respect, and ask him or her to express his or her thoughts and feelings. Here are some things you should *not* try:

- Do not try to force your ideas onto your adolescent and order her to follow your wishes.
- Do not scream or threaten to punish your child if he does not follow your advice.
- Do not try to win arguments for your ego's sake. Accept the fact that you need your adolescent child's consent to ensure her long-term success. Offer words that express your confidence in her ability to make the right decisions.

Referral to Weight-Management Centers

If you have an unmotivated or resistant obese adolescent, you may need advice from your child's doctor to find weight-management options in your area. Some teenagers need referral to a multidisciplinary weight-management center where trained counselors are available. In some cases, counseling with a child psychologist or psychiatrist may help adolescents to understand their emotional and weight issues. For adolescents who do not make progress controlling their weight at home, with family support or under medical supervision, bariatric surgery may be an option (see chapter 11).

Symptoms and Signs of Complications of Obesity

Common complications of obesity (discussed in chapter 1) include high cholesterol levels (hypercholesterolemia), hypertension, liver dysfunction, early signs of diabetes, hypertriglyceridemia, metabolic syndrome, and so on. The diagnosis of hypertension requires blood pressure measurements by your child's doctor. Other conditions require laboratory tests to make the diagnosis.

Less common complications can affect almost every system in the body. Some important clinical symptoms and signs of some of these less common complications are briefly described below. You should be knowledgeable of the signs and promptly report your concerns to your child's doctor if you observe evidence of them. Some complications require immediate attention. Box 8.2 summarizes the signs that should alert you to possible complications and their causes.

Box 8.2 Symptoms that may suggest complications of obesity

SYMPTOMS	POSSIBLE CAUSES
Severe recurrent headache (this requires urgent investigation)	Pseudotumor cerebri
Snoring, apnea (i.e., transient cessation of breathing), daytime sleepiness	Obstructive sleep apnea Obesity hypoventilation syndrome
Shortness of breath, exercise intolerance	Asthma Lack of physical conditioning
Abdominal pain	Gastroesophageal reflux disease Nonalcoholic fatty liver disease (NAFLD) Gallbladder disease Constipation
Hip pain, knee pain, walking pain	Slipped capital femoral epiphysis Musculoskeletal stress from weight
Foot pain	Musculoskeletal stress from weight
Absent or irregular menses (fewer than 9 cycles per year)	Polycystic ovary syndrome
Polyuria (excessive urination) and polydypsia (excessive intake of water)	Type 2 diabetes
Unexpected weight loss	Type 2 diabetes
Nocturnal enuresis (bedwetting during the night)	Obstructive sleep apnea
Anxiety, school avoidance, and social isolation	Depression
Sleepiness or wakefulness	Depression

Modified from S. E. Barlow and the Expert committee, "Expert Committee recommendations regarding the prevention, assessment, and treatment of child and adolescent overweight and obesity: summary." *Pediatrics* 120 (2007): S164–S192).

Does Your Obese Child Have Severe Headaches?

If your child experiences severe headaches, bring this to the attention of your child's doctor. Severe headache, especially in association with vomiting, blurred vision or diplopia (double vision), reduced visual acuity, and photophobia (increased sensitivity to light), may indicate a condition called pseudotumor cerebri. This condition is extremely rare but serious. Clinical symptoms are similar to those of a brain tumor (thus the name). The causes are numerous, but it is more common in obese children. When this condition is suspected, it requires urgent referral to a neurology specialist for investigation and treatment. If diagnosis is delayed, permanent neurologic damage with visual impairment may occur.

Does Your Child Snore Loudly at Night?

If your child snores loudly, with pauses in breathing, and experiences restless sleep at night and daytime sleepiness, she needs to be evaluated for obstructive sleep apnea or obesity hypoventilation syndrome. Report these symptoms to your child's physician for evaluation. Diagnosis may require the use of polysomnography (PSG) or a sleep study. Polysomnography is a recording of the physiological changes that occur in the brain (electroencephalography), eye (electrooculography), skeletal muscle activity (electromyography), and heart rhythm (electrocardiography) during sleep. Weight loss will help the condition. Most children benefit from removing the tonsils and adenoids (adenotonsillectomy). Sometimes treatment of coexisting asthma and gastroesophageal reflux helps. Some children eventually require positive pressure ventilation to achieve adequate oxygenation during sleep. If left untreated, children can develop complications such as pulmonary hypertension, hypertension, and heart failure.

Does Your Child Exhibit Shortness of Breath and Exercise Intolerance?

If he or she does, your child may have asthma or be physically unfit. Bring this to your child's doctor's attention so that your child can be appropriately evaluated for asthma. If asthma has been ruled out, the signs may point to a poor level of fitness. Have your child gradually increase the length and intensity of physical activities to improve fitness.

Does Your Child Complain of Abdominal Pain?

If your child experiences abdominal pain (either intermittent or severe colicky pain), the following conditions should be considered: NAFLD, gallstones, gastroesophageal reflux disease (GERD), and constipation. Bring any severe abdominal pain complaints to the attention of your child's doctor for diagnostic work-up.

NAFLD, also known as hepatic steatosis (meaning fatty change or degeneration), describes a condition in which there is accumulation of fat in the liver of people who do not drink significant amounts of alcohol. NAFLD has been reported in 25–50 percent of very obese adolescents. Most people with the condition have no symptoms, but the condition is usually suspected when liver enzyme abnormalities are discovered during routine laboratory tests. Additional studies by ultrasound or computed tomography (CT) may be required for diagnosis. A definitive diagnosis is made by a liver biopsy. Hepatic steatosis alone may be benign and reversible when the cause is eliminated. Rarely, the benign condition may progress to nonalcoholic steatohepatitis (NASH), which is an advanced stage of the disease (additional inflammation and fibrosis with significant liver damage).

Gallstones may cause an "attack" that is characterized by steady, severe pain in the right upper abdomen. It can radiate to the right shoulder and last for thirty minutes or more. Gallstone attacks often follow fatty meals, and they may occur at night. An ultrasound scan can produce images of gallstones without risks.

GERD is caused by dysfunction of the ring muscle, at the lower end of the esophagus, which allows stomach acid back into the esophagus, causing irritation or injury. It occurs more frequently in obese children than in nonobese children. Symptoms may include heartburn, vomiting, or pain with swallowing.

Children with severe constipation may experience symptoms such as bloating, distension, abdominal pain, or a sense of incomplete emptying. In obese children, constipation is due to inactivity and lack of fiber in the diet.

Does Your Child Complain of Leg or Foot Pain?

Overweight children more frequently complain of pain in the knee, ankles, and groin due to the extra weight they are carrying. They experience a greater frequency of fractures. They also show a greater frequency of misalignment of their lower extremities, which causes their lower legs to angle inward (Blount disease). Complaints of lower-limb pain may signal conditions that require orthopedic consultation and treatment. Pain in the hip, groin, thigh, or knee and pain with walking are symptoms of a condition called slipped capital femoral epiphysis. In this condition, the ball at the upper end of the femur (thigh bone) slips off in a backward direction. Most often, it develops during adolescence, and 50–70 percent of patients with the condition are obese. An X-ray confirms the diagnosis. Treatment is surgical pinning of the hip. If your child complains of pain or discomfort in the legs or feet on walking, consult your child's physician or an orthopedic surgeon, as lack of attention can lead to permanent injury to bones and joints.

Does Your Obese Daughter Have Irregular Menstrual Periods?

Infrequent menses (fewer than nine cycles per year) is the most important indication that your daughter may have polycystic ovary syndrome. This condition is due to an imbalance in hormones, with an excessive amount of male hormones (androgens) in genetically susceptible females. Untreated, it may lead to complications such as high blood pressure, heart problems, and diabetes as well as future difficulties getting pregnant. It occurs more often in obese women ages eighteen to twenty-five. They may have hirsutism (excessive and increased hair growth), excessive acne, and acanthosis nigricans, and they often develop type 2 diabetes. When such signs and symptoms are present, your daughter needs to be evaluated by an endocrinologist or gynecologist.

Psychological Issues That May Jeopardize Weight-Control Efforts

Besides sneaking food and bullying, other serious issues may jeopardize weight-loss efforts. These may include depression, eating disorders, trying diet pills, and wanting to have weight-loss surgery.

Depression

Depression frequently accompanies obesity in children. Flat affect, anxiety, body dissatisfaction, excessive eating, fatigue, and difficulty sleeping are some of the symptoms. A family history of depression increases the chances that a child may become depressed. A recent review found evidence that obesity causes depression and depression exacerbates obesity, which means that the cycle must be broken as part of any successful weight-loss program (Reeves et al. 2008, 103–114). Depressed people have more difficulty adhering to weight-management plans because of difficulty adhering to a fitness regimen, overeating, and negative thoughts. Dieting can worsen mood. Some antidepressants can cause weight gain. Doctors can administer a brief depression inventory to determine whether your child has mood disturbances as well as their severity. In some cases, depression may be accompanied by suicidal thoughts, indicating an acute psychiatric emergency.

Eating Disorders

If your overweight teenager concludes that his attempts at sensible weight-loss efforts are not working, he might move from one fad diet to another with nothing to show for it but anguish and frustration. She might resort to an eating disorder like bulimia nervosa or anorexia nervosa. About 1 percent of the female population in the United States has anorexia, and 1–4 percent has bulimia. About 1 percent of obese children and adolescents have bulimia nervosa; anorexia nervosa is much less frequent than bulimia. Most eating disorders occur in females (only about 10 percent in males). Be on the lookout for signs of eating disorders. If you suspect one, your child's doctor will probably refer your child to a specialist or treatment facility in this field. Your teenager is not likely to outgrow an eating disorder without professional help, so get it as early as possible.

Bulimia nervosa is characterized by bingeing on food (often high-calorie junk food), consuming thousands of calories over an hour or two, and purging by self-induced vomiting or abuse of laxatives or diuretics. Bulimics often hide food in their dresser drawers or closet. Behaviors that may be noticed include compulsive exercising, discarded packages for laxatives, diet pills, emetics (drugs that induce vomiting), or diuretics (drugs that reduce fluids, also called water pills), regularly going to the bathroom right after meals, and suddenly eating large amounts of food or buying large quantities of food that disappear right away. The weight fluctuates within a normal range. Bulimics may become depressed or experience severe mood swings. The prognosis of bulimia is much better than for anorexia nervosa.

Anorexia nervosa is characterized by the refusal to maintain a healthy body weight and an obsessive fear of gaining weight. Persons with anorexia nervosa continue to feel hunger but deny themselves all but small quantities of food. About 50 percent of patients with anorexia have symptoms of bulimia. It is a serious mental illness with a high incidence of complications in every organ system, and it has the highest mortality rate of any psychiatric disorder. The extreme dieting and weight loss can lead to heart rhythm disturbances, digestive abnormalities, bone density loss, anemia, hormonal and electrolyte imbalances, and a potentially fatal degree of malnutrition. The prognosis of anorexia is variable—some people make a full recovery, but others do not.

Diet Pills and Surgery

While long-lasting, effective weight-control programs take time to establish, in a society that promotes unrealistic body ideals and values the quick fix, it is not surprising that some obese teenagers turn to diet pills or think about surgery as the solution to their weight problem.

Some teenagers try over-the-counter pills or herbal products that promise to melt away the pounds with no effort. While such promises are enticing, they are hollow, as no pill melts away fat. You should never use medications on your own. Although medication is acceptable in order to achieve weight loss in some cases, and in combination with the methods described in this book, they should be used only under a physician's supervision to monitor nutrition and side effects. Two medications currently approved for use in the management of adolescent obesity are Xenical (orlistat) and Meridia (sibutramine). The former works by limiting absorption of fat, and the latter works by suppressing hunger sensations and increasing metabolic rate (see chapter 11).

Some obese teenagers want surgery as a quick answer rather than a long, slow lifestyle change. It should be pointed out to all children and their parents that even though surgical operations can have dramatic weight-loss benefits, they are not without risks, and the long-term effects and safety for adolescents are not completely understood. Even after surgery, obese teenagers still have to change the way they eat and exercise. Current national guidelines recommend surgery only for those patients with severe obesity and obesity-related complications. Even in those cases, surgery is performed only after a trial period of lifestyle change (at least six months) through a weight-management clinic (see chapter 11).

CASE 4

JC was a 14-year-old boy brought to the weight management clinic by his mother. JC was the only child in an East Asian family. His father was a successful restaurant owner and worked long hours. He had limited contact with JC, and even less influence on him. The family lived in an upper middle class neighborhood and JC was provided with everything he wanted.

JC was moderately obese. His unhealthy lifestyles included watching too many hours of television and spending hours on his computers, not spending much time outside, and eating too much fast food. He did not like to play outside with the neighborhood children. JC's mother bought him a bicycle as well as roller blades and encouraged him to use them, but JC did not use them regularly.

During JC's first visit to the weight management clinic, educational counseling reviewed the basics of obesity including its causes, complications, and treatment. During the discussion, JC's mother frequently interjected and blamed JC for not doing what she asked him to do to stay active. JC always responded by arguing and making excuses, and the arguments continued for long periods of time. JC complained his mother nags him about everything, and his mother blamed him for not following her recommendations. When the time for setting goals came, JC did not say much and his mother made most of the decisions. When seen on follow-ups, it was clear that JC did not make any attempt to achieve the goals set by his mother, and his mother continued to blame and scold him during the interviews. The same sequence of events occurred when JC's cholesterol level was found to be elevated.

After 3 return visits, it was clear that JC was not making any effort to adhere to the weight low program, and it was mutually agreed by the clinic staff and JC's mother that he should not return to the counseling sessions. Instead, it was suggested that he (and his mother) be seen by a pediatric psychologist to see if his attitude could be changed. Initially, JC and his mother resisted the suggestion, but given the lack of improvement in JC's weight status, they eventually agreed to attend several sessions with a pediatric psychologist, both separate and together. Through these sessions, both JC and his mother have made remarkable changes in their relationship and they were encouraged to return to the weight clinic. When they returned 6 months later, the encounters had changed dramatically; JC's mother did not interject and JC was more communicative and pleasant. Within 6 months of follow-up, JC showed signs of improvement with a significant reduction in his BMI.

This illustrates a case in which the parent-adolescent conflict was the major barrier against advancing the weight control effort. JC's mother admitted that she was treating him the same way as when he was a little boy; however, during their sessions with the psychologist she came to realize that her method of communicating with her adolescent son would not aid them in JC's weight loss program, she resolved to redefine the way they interacted in such a way to allow JC to express his own wishes.

Chapter 9

At the Destination

Your child has reached the destination of his long journey to a healthy weight goal. Congratulations! You must be very happy and proud of your child's accomplishment. However, do not celebrate as if your child finished a forty-kilometer marathon. It doesn't mean your child can stop her healthy routine. Even though your child's weight has reduced to a healthy level (the 85th percentile BMI), vigilance should be maintained until the healthy behaviors become routine for everybody in the family.

It is highly likely that your child will experience ups and downs as her life circumstances change, and you need to remain vigilant and continue to monitor your child and family for possible missteps.

Stage 6 of Prochaska's stages of change involves either maintenance or relapse. Relapse is frequent in any type of lifestyle change, including smoking cessation and rehabilitation from drug or alcohol addiction. Risk factors for relapse include the following:

- Despite successful weight control, your child may still have unhealthy behaviors. The newly acquired healthy behaviors can vanish and take your child right back to where he started.
- Family members who have not arrived at their weight goals or have remaining unhealthy behaviors can spoil your child's success.

Strategies to Prevent Relapse

Three strategies are recommended to help prevent relapse:

- Set new goals and try to reach those goals through behavior change.
- Continue self-monitoring the healthy behaviors.
- Check the BMI and risk factors regularly if less frequently.

1. Set New Goals

To maintain a healthy weight, your child needs to maintain his or her new healthy lifestyle. One of the fastest ways to relapse is to break his or her routine. Simply trying to maintain a healthy lifestyle often is not enough. Setting new goals, just as he or she did in the past, may be a better way. Your child can work on unhealthy behaviors that have not yet been corrected or further improve new healthy behaviors.

a. Uncorrected Unhealthy Behaviors

Even if your child has reached the target weight, he or she will undoubtedly have unhealthy behaviors that have not been fully corrected. Even nonobese individuals have unhealthy behaviors that could be improved.

- Your child might have reached a healthy weight by focusing on healthy eating behaviors but not incorporated adequate physical activity into his daily routine. Continue efforts to help him reach a healthy level of physical activity.

- Reduction in screen time may not be adequately addressed despite initial progress. If your child is still spending more than two hours watching TV, working on a computer, or playing electronic games, she can set new goals to reduce screen time further.

- Your child may be eating too many fast-food meals and not enough fruits and vegetables. New goals for increased consumption of fruits and vegetables should be made.

b. Improve New Healthy Behaviors

- If your child is now exercising for one hour every day, you may ask her to increase the time to more than an hour or increase the intensity.

- Although your child started exercising to burn calories, he may now enjoy it for its own sake. Encourage him to work toward improving skills at that activity, which will simultaneously encourage him to exercise for longer periods.

- Encourage your child to take up a new sport. It could be swimming, basketball, tennis, baseball, football, cross-country running, and so on. This can be a whole new world of challenges.

2. Continue Self-Monitoring of Healthy Behaviors

While your child continues working toward her new goals, continue to monitor her health behaviors on a regular basis as you did in the past (discussed in chapter 7). The importance of the child-parent interaction remains critical. It provides opportunities to examine and reflect on your efforts. You may now decide to review healthy behaviors with your child without using the form, as in the past, though you should still have these interactions at least once a week.

There are two ways to review healthy behaviors.

a. The 5-2-1-0 message plus moderation of SoFAS or FFC

Go over the 5-2-1-0 message at least once a week. Check whether your child is living according to the recommended healthy lifestyle (discussed in chapters 1 and 10).

- Is your child eating enough fruits and vegetables? Aim for five cups of fruits and vegetables a day. This will naturally reduce the consumption of high-energy-density food. Remind yourself of MyPlate, in which half the plate is filled with fruits and vegetables.
- Is your child watching TV, playing electronic games, or working on a computer for more than two hours a day?
- Is your child staying active and exercising for more than one hour every day?
- Is your child drinking regular sodas or sugary drinks?

One of the following two concepts completes your review of weight-control targets: "Moderation of SoFAS" and "Moderation of FFC." FFC stands for Fast food, Fried food, and Chips. These phrases are especially important if your child is not eating five cups of fruits and vegetables a day. As discussed earlier, SoFAS stands for solid fat and added sugar (and salt). Alternatively, you can refer to the "Moderation of FFC" message. The goal of that message is limiting consumption of high-fat food.

b. Healthy lifestyle checklists

The second option is to use the reminder presented in box 9.1. It is more or less a complete list of what this book has advised to control your child's weight problem.

3. Checking Your Child's Weight Status and Risk Factors

Even after your child has reached the target goal, check your child's and family members' weight occasionally (e.g., every month) to make sure that they have not gained significant amounts of weight. Your child is expected to gain weight as she grows, but excessive gain should alert you to a possible relapse. Calculate his BMI and the percentile value. This is a reliable way to check for relapse. If your child experiences a relapse, immediately return to the weight-management efforts and take the appropriate steps to deal with the relapse (see "Setbacks" in chapter 8).

To obtain an independent assessment of your child's health, have your child's doctor check on her general health, blood pressure, cholesterol, triglycerides, glucose, liver enzymes, and other issues on a yearly or semiannual basis.

Box 9.1. Checklist of healthy lifestyle behaviors

FOR THE CHILD	
	Being physically active for more than sixty minutes every day, including school PE time
	Limiting screen time (TV viewing, working on computers, and electronic games) to less than two hours a day
	Aim for five ounces of fruits and vegetables a day. Use fruits and vegetables for main dishes and use them as snacks
	No regular soft drinks or fruit drinks ____ Limit orange juice to no more than one glass a day
	Reduce the frequency of eating fast food, including school lunches (if they remain unhealthy) as much as possible
	Reduce the consumption of fried food, fast food, French fries, and chips
	Other behavioral changes ____ Switch to 1% or skim milk ____ Switch to whole-wheat bread ____ No skipping breakfast ____ No snacks after-dinner (within three hours of bedtime) ____ No TV viewing while eating

FOR THE PARENTS	
	Buying more fruits and vegetables. Remember five servings a day ____ Make more main meals with vegetables ____ Vegetable and fruit snacks?
	Serve more whole-grain products such as cereals, breads, and others
	Do not buy regular high-fat and/or high-sugar snacks such as chips, ice creams, cakes, and cookies ____ Not keeping unhealthy snacks in the house
	Do not buy regular dairy products, including cheeses. Buy low-fat or fat-free products
	Buying lean meat, poultry, and fish, and trimming off visible fat before cooking
	Do not pan fry or deep fry food when cooking
	Do not buy or serve too much potato
	Regularly check nutrition facts lable
	Reduce frequency of eating restaurant food, including the take-out food
	Have healthy family dinner often
	Have family outings during the weekend

Part 2

Advanced Knowledge in Obesity

Part 2 provides an advanced knowledge base, beyond that necessary to carry out the home-based weight-management efforts for your child. In this part, a number of obesity-related topics are discussed in detail. These range from pedometer use, the concepts of energy balance, "good" fat and "bad" fat, and the glycemic index, how to read the nutrition facts labels, and finally to surgical approaches for severe obesity.

The information provided in this part probably represents more than that offered by weight-clinic staff. The knowledge gained, though, will give you a sound scientific understanding of the approaches used in part 1. In addition, information here can be used to help friends and relatives who have similar weight problems with their children.

Chapter 10

Advanced Topics in Obesity

This chapter is primarily for parents who want additional information, have unanswered questions from chapter 5, or want to be able to advise friends or relatives with similar weight problems. Reading this chapter before initiating actual weight-management efforts is not necessary, because chapter 5 provides sufficient information to proceed.

Pedometers

Pedometers are electronic or electromechanical devices worn at the hip to count the number of steps walked per day, giving an estimate of the distance walked. Today's pedometers are small, relatively inexpensive, and user-friendly, and they can serve as a wonderful motivator for meeting the daily recommended goal for steps taken (a measurement of overall physical activity). Start with a simple pedometer that counts steps and has a reset button.

Pedometers have been used to set a measurable goal of walking in adults and children, and show some success in controlling weight gain. Using a pedometer may be a helpful way of self-monitoring physical activity. A recent meta-analysis of studies involving 2,767 obese adult patients showed that wearing a pedometer increased the physical activity of the average subject by more than two thousand steps (approximately one mile) per day, along with a concurrent significant decrease in BMI and blood pressure (Bravata et al. 2007, 296–304). It appears that setting a step goal and recording it in a step diary may be a key motivational factor for increasing physical activity. For an obese individual, the beginning step goal may be set low, then gradually increased to the recommended level.

The recommended steps per day are as follows:

- For adults: A goal of ten thousand steps is common for adults, based on its adoption by walking clubs and representations by pedometer companies in Japan promoting its use. This is the equivalent of about five miles. It may seem like a lot, but if you count all the steps you take in daily activities, at work, and at home doing chores, they might be more than you realize. Adults who want to lose weight should strive for fifteen to twenty thousand steps per day. (There is no body of research to back up that number, though.) Note that two thousand adult steps is equivalent to about one mile, which for adults burns about 100 Calories.
- For children: Emerging data indicate that ten thousand steps is likely to be too low a number to elicit substantial health benefits. Laurson and colleagues recommend thirteen thousand steps per day for boys, eleven thousand per day for girls, and twelve thousand per day for both sexes combined as pedometer guidelines for children in the United States (Laurson et al. 2008, 419–424). Obese children may need more steps to lose weight.

Are Pedometers Accurate?

The accuracy of step counters varies widely between devices. The best pedometers are accurate to within about 5 percent. Typically, step counters are reasonably accurate at a walking pace on a flat surface if the device is placed in its optimal position (usually vertically on the belt clip). An accelerometer, which is worn at the ankle, is a more sophisticated research tool. It measures the acceleration of movement in three directions: up/down, right/left, and forward/backward. It also measures the distance walked and estimates the total energy expended, but it is expensive and requires expertise to use. When it comes to encouraging people to be physically active, pedometers are still useful in setting goals for physical activity.

Detailed Energy Balance Equation

The energy balance considered in chapter 1 is not adequate to understand the role of exercise in weight control. Energy expenditure is more complicated than that shown in fig. 1.1. Figure 10.1 breaks down energy intake and expenditure as we understand them now.

The source of energy (left side of the balance) is what we eat, including carbohydrates, proteins, and fat. Fat is the most energy-dense food, providing 9 kcal (Calorie) per gram, while proteins and carbohydrates provide 4 kcal (Calorie) per gram.

There are three components of energy expenditure (right side of the balance): physical activity, thermal effect of food (TEF), and RMR.

- RMR accounts for a large portion of energy expenditure, some 60–75 percent. RMR is the amount of energy expended at complete rest for functioning of the vital organs like the heart, lungs, liver, kidneys, and so on. Even during sleep, a large amount of energy is burned.

- Approximately 10 percent of energy is dispatched through the TEF, which mainly results from the energy cost involved in nutrient absorption, processing, and storage.

- It is noteworthy that energy expenditure resulting from physical activity is much smaller than the RMR, accounting for 10–20 percent of total energy expenditure.

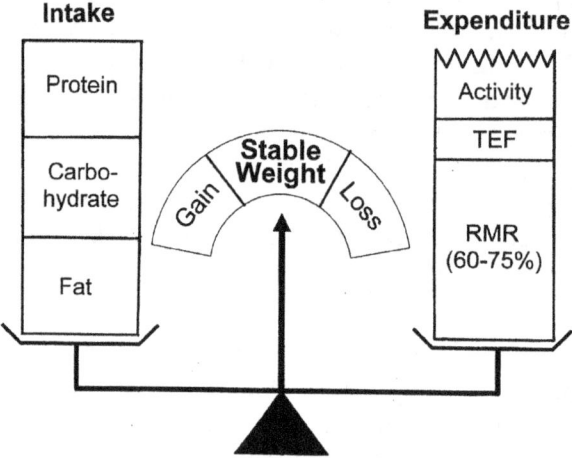

Figure 10.1. Detailed energy balance. When intake exceeds expenditure, weight gain occurs. When expenditure exceeds intake, weight loss may result. Note that a relatively small portion of energy expenditure results from physical activities. Reproduced by permission from Myung K. Park, *Park's Pediatric Cardiology for Practitioners*, 6th ed. (Philadelphia: Mosby, 2014).

Energy expenditures from RMR and TEF may be determined by genetic factors, and they stay relatively constant. Energy expenditure from physical activity varies greatly from individual to individual. The only component of energy expenditure that can be changed is physical activity.

Ways to Lose Weight Based on the Energy Balance Equation

According to the energy balance equation, body weight remains stable in adults when caloric intake equals caloric expenditure. In growing children, calorie intake should be larger than expenditure to allow for normal growth. There are three ways to lose weight by "unbalancing" the energy balance equation (fig. 10.1):

- Reduce caloric intake below the daily requirements
- Increase energy expenditure through additional physical activity while maintaining normal caloric intake
- Combine both methods, which is more effective than one method alone

Why Is It Difficult to Lose Weight by Reducing Energy Intake Alone?

You may lose weight by eating a severely calorie-restricted diet alone, but the success is usually short lived, and you eventually regain the weight. Weight loss that occurs from dieting is accompanied by a dramatic reduction in RMR (as much as 45 percent). In this case, exercise tends to increase metabolic rate and opposes the body's tendency to maintain the current weight. Weight control is more successful when you combine reduced calorie intake with increased physical activity.

Why Is Regular Exercise Important in Reducing Weight?

Research emphasizes exercise as a component of weight-control strategies:

- It uses calories that would otherwise be stored as fat.
- It counteracts the body's response of lowering RMR when calories are reduced.
- It increases RMR, the major component of energy expenditure, by nearly 10 percent.
- Even after exercising, energy expenditure remains high for up to seven hours.

Diet-induced weight loss results in the reduction of not only body fat but also fat-free mass, such as muscle. Regular exercise retards lean-tissue loss and conserves, even increases, fat-free body mass.

Examples of Calories Burned during Exercise

Calories burned vary with the weight of the person exercising, because it takes more energy to move larger objects. The heavier the person, the more calories burned per unit time for the same activity. Table 10.1 shows the approximate number of calories spent per hour by persons of varying weights for the activities listed. Note that a person weighing 100 lb. needs to walk for one hour at a slow pace to burn the calories in a 12 oz. can of regular soda.

Table 10.1 Physical activity calorie use chart

ACTIVITY (1 HOUR)	BODY WEIGHT		
	100 lb.	150 lb.	200 lb.
Bicycling, 6 mph	160	240	312
Bicycling, 12 mph	270	410	534
Jogging, 7 mph	610	920	1,230
Jump roping	500	750	1,000
Running, 5.5 mph	440	660	962
Running, 10 mph	850	1,280	1,664
Swimming, 25 yards/min.	185	275	358
Swimming, 50 yards/min.	325	500	650
Tennis singles	265	400	535
Walking, 2 mph (slow pace)	160	240	312
Walking, 3 mph (moderate pace)	210	320	416
Walking, 4.5 mph (very brisk pace)	295	440	572

The American Heart Association, "Physical activity calorie use chart." (2010). [http://www.healthy-firefighter.org/fitness/physical-activity-calorie-use-chart.

Don't reward your child with a "treat" for calories burned during exercise. People generally overestimate the calories burned during exercise and reward themselves with excess calories, thereby creating a net gain in calories consumed.

Glycemic Index and Glycemic Load

Glycemic index (GI) has become an important concept in the field of obesity research. Several decades ago, the US government, the AHA, and other scientific organizations recommended that people eat low-fat diets to reduce weight gain and improve cardiovascular health. However, low-fat diets have not always been successful in reducing weight gain and improving cardiovascular risk status. Moreover, mean fat intake in the United States has decreased since the 1960s (from 42 to 34 percent of dietary energy), yet the prevalence of obesity has risen in the last several decades. During the same period, an increase in carbohydrate consumption has been observed (Brand-Miller et al. 2002, 281S–285S).

Low-fat diets were usually high in carbohydrates, making up for lost calories from fat, and therefore in this case people were eating low-fat/high-carbohydrate diets. On the other hand, low-carbohydrate diets (with more protein and fat), such as the Atkins diet, eventually became popular, appearing to be effective in terms of weight reduction. Researchers started asking why a low-fat/high-carbohydrate diet did not work well but a high-fat/low-carbohydrate diet seemed to work for some people. They suspected that some of the carbohydrates may not be good thing in controlling weight, and they started looking at the *quality* of the carbohydrates in low-fat diets. It turned out that the carbohydrates consumed by people on low-fat diets were mostly refined and high in sugar content (i.e., high-GI food) (Ludwig et al. 1999, E261–E266; Brand-Miller et al. 2002, 281S–285S).

Glycemic Index

The concept of GI was described by Dr. David J. Jenkins of the University of Toronto and his colleagues in 1981 to express the rapidity with which a carbohydrate diet is digested and absorbed into the bloodstream (Jenkins et al. 1981, 362–366). All carbohydrates are not created equal. Even with equal amounts of total carbohydrate, some foods cause a higher and quicker rise in blood sugar than others. It was incorrectly assumed that a complex carbohydrate like starch, which has a higher number of glucose molecules joined by chemical bonds, was absorbed more slowly than simple sugars such as glucose and table sugar. That assumption was wrong; the number of glucose molecules in a complex carbohydrate like starch was determined not to be important in the rate of digestion and absorption. White bread and baked potato, which are rich in starch, were digested and absorbed as quickly as table sugar (sucrose).

The GI is the number given to a food based on how quickly it raises blood sugar levels. Following ingestion of enough food to provide 50 gm of a particular carbohydrate, blood glucose levels are determined and plotted every fifteen minutes for the first hour and every thirty minutes for the second hour (for a total of two hours). The area under the resulting curve is calculated. The same is done following ingestion of 50 gm of glucose, and the area under the curve is again calculated. The area under the curve for a particular food and that for glucose are then compared with the index of pure glucose set at 100. GI is classified as follows:

- A GI of 55 or less is low.
- A GI of 55–69 is medium (or intermediate).
- A GI of 70 or more is high.

GI applies only to foods that contain carbohydrates; it is less important or not relevant to foods with mostly fat and protein. Examples of low-, medium-, and high-GI foods are shown in table 10.2.

Table 10.2 Classification of glycemic index and examples

CLASSIFI-CATION	GI RANGE	EXAMPLES
Low GI	55 or less	Most fruits and vegetables (except potatoes), whole-grain products, legumes, whole-grains, nuts and seeds, and fructose
Medium GI	56—69	Whole-wheat products, stone-ground breads, whole-grain cereal, table sugar, some brown rice, sweet potato, corn taco shells, and some cakes and cookies
High GI	70 or more	White bread, baked potatoes, some processed cereals, most white rice, cornflakes, most muffins, honey, some cookies and cakes, most food made with enriched white floor, watermelon, and glucose

Here is some general information about the GI of various foods:

- In general, fruits, vegetables (except potatoes), and legumes have a low GI, while sweets, refined-grain products (e.g., white bread), and potatoes have a high GI.
- The presence of fat lowers the GI. A baked potato has a GI of 85, but fried potatoes (French fries) have a GI of 75.
- The presence of soluble dietary fiber lowers the GI. Whole-wheat breads with higher amounts of fiber generally have a lower GI than white breads.
- The way food is prepared can change its GI. A boiled potato has a GI of 56, steamed potatoes have a GI of 65, and a microwaved potato has a GI of 82.
- The ripeness of fruit increases the GI. The GI of underripe bananas is 30, while that of overripe bananas is 52.
- Organic acids or their salts (e.g., adding vinegar) lowers the GI.

Glycemic Load

One criticism of the GI is that it tells only how rapidly 50 g of carbohydrate in a particular food turns into blood sugar, but it does not tell how much of that carbohydrate is in a serving of a particular food. The glycemic load (GL) is a new way of assessing the impact of carbohydrate consumption that takes into account serving size. For example, although candies have a high GI, eating a single piece of candy, which contains a small fraction of 50 g, will result in a relatively small glycemic response. Thus, the GL of the candy is not high. The carbohydrate in watermelon has a high GI (72), but watermelon's glycemic load is low (4 from 120 g of watermelon).

A GL of a typical serving of food is the product of the amount of available carbohydrate in that serving and the GI of the food (calculated by the amount of carbohydrate contained in a specified serving size of the food x the GI of that food ÷ 100). For a single meal, for example:

- A GL of ≥ 20 points is considered high.
- A GL of 11 to 19 points is medium.
- A GL of ≤ 10 points is low.

The higher the food's GL, the greater the expected elevation in blood glucose after consumption. A diet with a low GL has been linked to a lower risk of heart disease. A diet low in carbohydrate automatically has a low glycemic load. Almost all food with a low GI has a low GL.

Glycemic Index and Glycemic Load for Selected Foods

Table 10.3 shows the GI and GL of selected foods. A more complete list of GI is periodically published by the American Society for Clinical Nutrition. The official website for glycemic index is http://www.ajcn.org/content/76/1/5.full.

Additional websites on GI and GL include http://www.mendosa.com/gilists.htm and http://www.glycemicindex.com.

Table 10.3 Glycemic index and glycemic load for selected foods*

FOOD	GI	GL†	FOOD	GI	GL†
Instant rice	91	24.8 (110 g)	Banana	53	13.3 (170 g)
Baked potato	85	20.3 (110 g)	Corn tortilla	52	12 (50 g)
Cornflakes	81	21 (30 g)	Wheat breads	50	10 (30 g)
French fries	75	22 (150 g)	Brown rice	50	16 (150 g)
Bagel, white	72	25 (70 g)	Orange	48	5 (120 g)
Carrot	71	3.6 (55 g)	Spaghetti	41	16.4 (55 g)
White bread	70	21.0 (2 slices)	Apple	36	8.1 (170 g)
Rye bread	65	19.5 (2 slices)	Lentil beans	29	5.7 (110 g)
Coca-Cola	63	16 (250 g)	Milk	27	3.2 (225 mL)
Sweet corn	60	11 (80 g)	Peanuts	14	0.7 (30 g)

* From various sources. The GI values vary somewhat from report to report.
† The numbers in the parentheses indicate the amount of the food consumed.
GI, glycemic index; GL, glycemic load.

How Does GI Relate to Weight Gain?

Dr. David S. Ludwig and his colleagues at Harvard University provided important information regarding hormonal and metabolic changes following ingestion of high- and low-GI diets in adolescents. The study renders how high-GI diets may cause early cravings for food and may contribute to weight gain.

Figure 10.2 shows the data reported by Ludwig and his colleagues:

- After consumption of a high-GI food, blood levels of glucose and insulin rose rapidly to much higher levels and stayed elevated for a longer period of time than seen in the low-GI food group (upper-right and upper-left panels).

- Blood levels of glucagon dropped markedly in the high-GI food group, but it increased markedly in the low-GI food group and remained so for four to five hours (lower-left panel).

- Several hours later, blood fatty acid and glucose levels were lower in the high-GI food group than in the low-GI food group (lower-right and upper-left panels, respectively).

- There was an increase in serum growth hormone levels four hours after the high-GI food (not shown), which may promote weight gain.

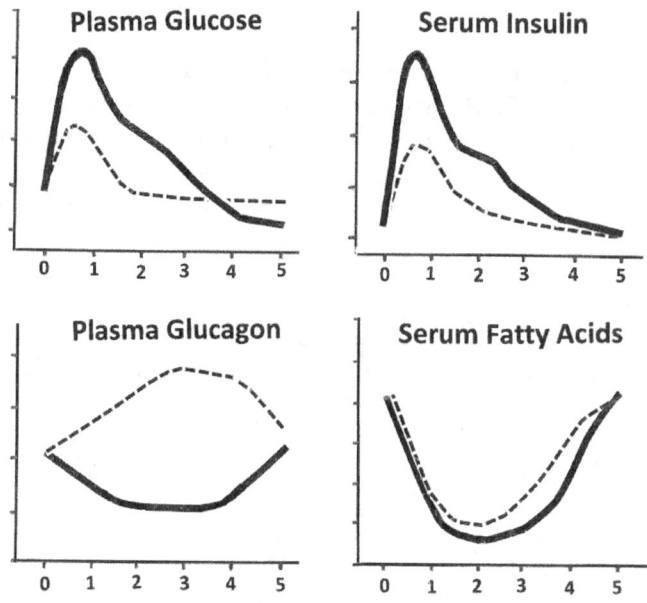

Figure 10.2. Comparison of hormonal and metabolic changes following ingestion of high-GI and low-GI food in adolescents. Tick lines represent the high-GI food group, and thin broken lines represent the low-GI food group. Redrawn from D. S. Ludwig et al., "High Glycemic Index Food, Overeating, and Obesity," *Pediatrics* (1999).

How May High-GI Diet Contributes to Weight Gain?

In the above study, two important differences were observed in blood glucose and serum fatty acid levels. Following consumption of a high-GI food, there were lower plasma glucose levels (four hours after eating) and lower levels of serum fatty acid (two hours after eating). These findings may offer partial explanation for weight gain following consumption of high-GI food through these possible mechanisms:

- Low glucose levels seen four hours after eating high-GI foods (reactive hypoglycemia) may trigger hunger sensations and lead to overeating, resulting in weight gain.
- Lower levels of serum fatty acid (two hours after eating) may mean that insulin forced fat cells to take in blood lipids (fatty acids) or a low level of glucagon impaired the breakdown of lipids (lipolysis) in the fat cells.
- The combined action of high insulin and low glucagon may be fat accumulation and preservation, resulting in weight gain.
- A higher level of growth hormone after eating a high-GI food (not shown in fig. 10.2) may also promote weight gain.

After eating a low-GI food, the levels of glucose and insulin are much lower, reactive hypoglycemia is not seen, and fatty acid levels remain higher, which may mean that lipids are not forced into the body cell or that high levels of glucagon made the cells break down fats and made more fatty acids available for the energy system.

What Is Glucagon?

Glucagon is a pancreatic hormone that increases blood glucose levels, opposite to the action of insulin. The major effect of glucagon is breakdown of liver glycogen (glycogenolysis), which increases blood glucose level within minutes. Glucagon activates adipose cell lipase (lipolysis), making more fatty acids available for the energy system.

Why Are High-GI or High-GL Foods Unhealthy?

Consuming high-GI food is unhealthy for several reasons:

- Reactive hypoglycemia resulting from high-GI food may promote food cravings and overeating, which contributes to weight gain.
- Low levels of fatty acids in high-GI food may suggest that fatty acids are taken into the fat cells or that breakdown of fat did not take place in the fat cells (by high levels of glucagon). Both lead to fat accumulation.
- High levels of blood glucose and insulin may predispose one to the development of diabetes.
- High-GI foods produce undesirable metabolic effects similar to those seen in metabolic syndrome, thus increasing the risk of developing heart disease. These include raising blood triglyceride levels, raising LDL cholesterol, and lowering levels of HDL cholesterol.

What Is Good about Low-GI Food?

Consumption of low-GI foods has been shown to have the following benefits, opposite those described for high-GI foods:

- Following consumption of low-GI food, people feel fuller, and hunger pangs are delayed.

- Low-GI food helps control weight by actions opposite to the effects of high-GI food. Putting obese children on a low-GI diet seems to enhance weight loss.

- Low-GI food results in low glucose and insulin levels, and it reduces the risk of developing diabetes.

- The prevalence of metabolic syndrome is lower in people eating low-GI foods.

- A low-GI diet lowers the risk of heart disease and stroke by reducing triglycerides and LDL cholesterol levels, increasing HDL cholesterol, and reducing plasminogen activator inhibitor, thereby preventing the risk of blood clot formation.

High Triglyceride Levels

For several decades, LDL cholesterol has been the primary target of reducing heart disease with the use of statin medication. Since the 1990s, raised triglycerides in blood have been incriminated as a risk factor for heart disease. Hypertriglyceridemia is now accepted as a cause of heart disease, independent of the levels of cholesterols. Besides being associated with heart disease and diabetes, it tends to increase coagulability (blood clot formation) and decreases fibrinolysis (breakdown of blood clots), thereby increasing the risk of stroke.

How Are Lifestyle Factors Related to High Triglycerides?

Excess calorie intake from foods and lack of adequate physical activity are the major causes of hypertriglyceridemia and obesity.

Triglyceride is a fancy name for fat. From a chemical point of view, a triglyceride is any combination of glycerol (glyceride) with three fatty acids. Most of the fats we eat, including butter, margarine, and oil, are all in triglyceride form. Because of the similarity in the chemical structure, we have known for some time that high fat consumption is the cause of high triglyceride levels in the blood. High consumption of saturated fat (found in red meat, butter, lard, ice cream, cheese, whole milk dairy products, and fatty hamburgers) and trans fat (found in stick margarines, some packaged baked goods, and potato and other chips) causes high triglyceride levels.

A less well-known source of hypertriglyceridemia is carbohydrate in food. Consumption of high-GI food containing large amounts of simple sugar is a more important cause of hypertriglyceridemia than fats in the diet. Diets that are low in fat and high in simple sugars markedly stimulate fatty acid synthesis from carbohydrate, which raises plasma triglycerides. According to the Harvard School of Public Health, carbohydrates have a greater impact on triglyceride levels than dietary fats (Hellerstein 2002, 33–40). It is important to know that the source of triglyceride in the blood is not just dietary fat but also carbohydrate (sugar). Any unused calories from carbohydrates or fats become triglycerides in the liver.

A good example of hypertriglyceridemia is seen in individuals with metabolic syndrome (discussed in chapter 2). These are obese individuals with a sedentary lifestyle who consume a large amount of simple sugars. Surprisingly, they have abnormal lipid patterns characterized by high triglyceride levels rather than high cholesterol levels. Their cholesterol levels are not elevated, but they have "small dense LDL particles," which are much worse in producing coronary artery plaque than the usual cholesterol. Most studies show that metabolic syndrome is associated with a doubling of heart disease and stroke risk and five times the risk of developing type 2 diabetes (Mattillo et al. 2010, 1113–1132).

Causes of Hypertriglyceridemia

Besides the consumption of high-fat and high-GI foods, obesity, and a sedentary lifestyle, other causes of hypertriglyceridemia include diabetes, alcohol, smoking, hypothyroidism, liver and kidney diseases, and insulin resistance as a component of metabolic syndrome. Among these, consumption of high-GI food may be most important cause of hypertriglyceridemia, particularly in obese individuals.

How to Help Prevent or Treat Hypertriglyceridemia

High triglyceride levels can be lowered or prevented by doing the following:

- Consume large quantities of low-GI foods, such as whole-grain products, fruit, and vegetables, and reduce consumption of high-GI foods, such as refined-grain products and sugary food. High-GI food may be a more important cause of hypertriglyceridemia than high-fat food.

- Reduce consumption of saturated fats (found in beef, lamb, pork, and whole milk dairy products) and trans fat (found in deep-fried food and store-bought cakes, cookies, and crackers). Consume more chicken, turkey, and fish, which are low in saturated fat. Use unsaturated fats such as olive or vegetable oil instead of butter or lard for cooking.

- Increase physical activity. You can lower triglyceride levels by getting at least thirty minutes of moderate-intensity exercise five days per week. Exercise lowers triglycerides and LDL cholesterol, and it boosts HDL cholesterol levels.

- Lose weight if you are overweight.

- Limit alcohol intake. Even small amounts of alcohol can have a dramatic impact on triglyceride levels in adults.

- Stop smoking. Smoking can increase triglyceride levels.

- Treat other illnesses that can cause hypertriglyceridemia, such as diabetes, kidney or liver disease, and hypothyroidism.

Excessive Sugar Intake

Added sugar is a major health concern. The most important source of added sugar is soft drinks, which account for approximately one-third of the sugar intake among Americans. According to a study reported in the *Journal of the American Dietetic Association*, food groups that contribute to added sugars in the American diet are soft drinks (33 percent), sugars and candy (16 percent), cakes, cookies, and pies (13 percent), fruit drinks like fruit "ades" and fruit punches (10 percent), and dairy desserts and milk products (9 percent) (Ervin et al. 2012).

Soft drinks may be responsible for the doubling of obesity in children in the United States over the last fifteen years. In the past four decades, consumption of sweetened beverages increased for all age groups with a resulting increase in total energy intake (Troiano et al. 2000, 1343S–1353S; Spear et al. 2007, S254–S288).

Soft drink companies spend billions on advertising, and in a recent year, soft drink companies grossed more than $57 billion in sales in the United States alone. They produce enough soda annually to provide 600 eight-ounce servings (or 37.5 gallons) for every man, woman, and child. Average Americans older than two years consume 132 Calories per day from soft drinks and the intake of the consumption of the soft drink rose 1,000 percent between 1970 and 1990 (Vartanian et al. 2007, 667–675).

Since the 1960s, the beverage industry has increased the serving size from a standard 6.5 oz. bottle to a 20 oz. bottle and more. At 7-Eleven stores, soft drinks come as Gulps (20 oz.), Big Gulps (30 oz.), Super Big Gulps (40 oz.), and Double Gulps (50 oz.), which are said to "quench even the most diabolical thirst."

In many fast-food restaurants, unlimited soft drink refills are allowed, resulting in enormous consumption of soft drinks.

Why Is Too Much Sugar Unhealthy?
Consumption of too much sugar is unhealthy for the following reasons:

- High sugar content in food and drinks provides extra calories, and these turn into fat, resulting in weight gain.
- Sugar raises blood sugar and insulin levels and keeps them high longer than normal (hyperinsulinemia). Insulin moves sugar from the circulation into the cells, and it may move circulating fat into fat cells, resulting in fat accumulation (weight gain). Obesity is a prime risk factor for type 2 diabetes, heart disease, stroke, and other chronic diseases.
- Sugar raises triglyceride levels. Hypertriglyceridemia is a component of metabolic syndrome and an independent risk factor for heart disease.
- Sugar kills the appetite for more nourishing food and may actually increase hunger, resulting in increased food intake.
- Sugar promotes tooth decay.

- Sweet foods and soft drinks lack important nutrients such as vitamins, minerals, fiber, and protein.

Sugar Allowance

Nutrition fact labels do not show the recommended daily allowance (RDA) for sugar. The Food Standards Agency and the WHO say that no more than 10 percent of total calories should come from processed sugar.

Ten percent of 2,000 Calories for a ten-year-old is 200 Calories or 50 g of sugar (1 g of sugar equals 4 Calories). For a ten-year-old child who needs 2,000 Calories a day, 50 g (12.5 teaspoons) of sugar is the daily allowance. For adolescent boys and young men who need 3,000 Calories a day, the daily allowance will be 75 g (about 19 teaspoons).

Compare this with the sugar content of 40 g in a 12 oz. can of soda, which contains 80 percent of the daily sugar allowance for a child. It may be wise to avoid food or drink with sugar content of 20 g in a serving, which is 30–40 percent of the daily sugar allowance. Food or drinks with 10 g or less sugar per serving provide 15–20 percent of the daily allowance.

Examples of High-Sugar Food

Table 10.4 lists the sugar content of selected sugary foods. This is not a comprehensive list, but is provided to bring your attention to the high sugar content of some favorite popular foods and drinks. Check the food label for the sugar content of your child's favorite food, and compare it with your child's daily allowance, which is 50 g (or 75 g).

Impact of Chronic Consumption of Soft Drinks

Let us consider the hypothetical impact of a 12 oz. can of soda, which provides 150 Calories. Brisk walking for thirty minutes, slow walking for sixty minutes, or dancing for thirty minutes will burn the calories in a can of soda. This means that a person who drinks, for example, three sodas a day should exercise two to three hours every day just to burn the calories in the soda. Most people do not have time for that much activity. If you don't burn the excess calories, they will end up as fat.

Approximately 3,500 unused Calories will become one pound of fat. If you consume one can of soda a day (150 Calories) and do not burn the calories, you accumulate an extra 1,500 Calories in ten days (or 4,500 extra Calories in a month, which is more than a pound of fat). You can see that if you continue to drink one can of soda every day and don't burn off the calories over a year, you will gain about 15 lb. of fat. It is clear that your child should not consume calories that she cannot burn. It is also easy to understand how excessive consumption of soft drinks could have caused obesity in this country.

Table 10.4 Added sugars in selected food

	ITEM (amount)	TOTAL CALORIES	SUGAR (in grams)	SUGAR (in teaspoons)
Sodas	Pepsi, wild cherry (12 oz.)	160	42	10.5
	Diet Pepsi (12 oz.)	0	0	0
	Seagram's Ginger Ale (12 oz.)	130	35	8.8
	Sprite (12 oz.)	140	39	9.8
	Coca-Cola (12 oz.)	140	39	9.8
	Coca-Cola, cherry (12 oz.)	150	41	10
	Diet Coke (12 oz.)	1	0	0
	Pepsi (12 oz.)	150	41	10
	Root Beer (12 oz.)	160	40	10
	Hershey's chocolate milk (8 oz.)	200	30	7.5
Fruit Drinks	Capri-Sun fruit drink (6.4 oz.)	90	22.5	5.6
	Hawaiian Punch (12 oz.)	120	23	5.75
	Hi-C fruit punch (6.75 oz.)	100	25	4.25
	Minute Maid juice beverage (ruby grapefruit) (8 oz.)	130	32	8
	Ocean Spray, cranberry (12 oz.)	200	50	12.5
	Sunny Delight (6.75 oz.)	88	22	5.5
Energy Drinks	Red Bull Energy Drink (8.3 oz.)	108	27	6.75
	Rockstar Energy Drink (8 oz.)	124	31	7.75
Ice Teas	Arizona Lemon Ice Tea (8 oz.)	90	24	6.0
	Snapple Lemon Ice Tea (8 oz.)	100	23	5.75
Fruit Juices	Apple juice (8 oz.)	120	26	6.5
	Orange juice (8 oz.)	110	24	6.0
Others	Fruit-flavored yogurt (6-ounce)	92	23	5.75
	Butterfinger crisp (2) (40 g.)	200	19	4.75
	Chocolate donut (1)	76	19	4.75
	Ding Dongs (2) (80 g.)	360	35	8.75
	Granola bar (1)	40	10	2.5
	Milky Way candy bar (2) (34 g.)	150	20	5
	Old-fashioned donut (1)	56	14	3.5
	Musketeers (3) (45 g.)	190	30	7.5
	Twinkie (1) (43 g.)	150	19	4.5

How to Reduce Sugar Intake

Unhealthy consequences of excessive sugar intake are numerous, as discussed above. Reducing sugar intake is about preserving your health. The following are some commonsense approaches to reduce sugar intake.

1. Reduce consumption of the following foods and drinks:

    a. Soft drinks of all kinds except for diet or sugar-free
    b. Fruit "ades" and drinks like fruit punch and lemonade
    c. Cakes, cookies, pies, and candies
    d. Dairy desserts like ice cream

2. Learn to identify foods and drinks with a high content of sugar by checking the nutrition facts label. Avoid food with a sugar content higher than 20 g per serving. This is about 40 percent of the daily allowance for children ten years of age and 27 percent of the daily allowance for adolescents.
3. For dessert, serve fruit instead of pie, cake, or ice cream.
4. When cooking, use less sugar than a recipe calls for.
5. If you use canned fruit, drain the syrup before serving.
6. During holidays, ration candy and other sugary (or fatty) treats, and get rid of the excess after one week.

Fructose Is a Major Health Concern

Until the 1980s, soft drinks were sweetened with refined sucrose or corn syrup. Today, nearly all soft drinks are sweetened with high-fructose corn syrup (HFCS) because of its lower cost. To produce HFCS, corn is milled to produce cornstarch, and the cornstarch is mixed with water and an enzyme to produce corn syrup. Corn syrup, which is entirely glucose, undergoes enzymatic processing to increase the fructose content. An increasing number of studies criticize HFCS as having possibly caused obesity, type 2 diabetes, heart disease, metabolic syndrome, hyperactivity, tooth decay, and a host of other problems (Schulze et al. 2004, 927–934). Some studies dispute these criticisms, but the majority of those are industry sponsored.

HFCS has been implicated as follows:

- It may play a major role in the obesity crisis.
- It may be a contributing cause of metabolic syndrome. High fructose consumption may cause insulin resistance, obesity, and elevated levels of triglycerides, leading to metabolic syndrome, which has been linked to type 2 diabetes. The mechanism by which excess fructose consumption leads to metabolic syndrome is poorly understood.
- It can cause an increase in atherogenic lipids that cause coronary heart disease, including high levels of triglycerides, low levels of HDL cholesterol, and smaller particle size of LDL cholesterol.
- It may cause NAFLD.
- It may cause hyperactive behaviors and tooth decay.

Dietary Fiber

Dietary fiber, sometime called roughage, is that part of plants that cannot be digested by the enzymes of the digestive tract. The term "fiber" is a misnomer, because many of the so-called dietary fibers are not fibers at all. Dietary fiber is not one substance. Many consist of a variety of substances, most of which are complex carbohydrates such as cellulose and other plant components like dextrin, inulin, lignin, waxes, and pectin. Food appearing fibrous, like lettuce, is not necessarily high in fiber. Dietary fiber is not a good source of calories, minerals, or vitamins.

Sources of Dietary Fiber

Fiber is present in food derived from plants, including the following:

- Fruits (apples, pears, oranges, strawberries, and others)
- Vegetables (cabbage, broccoli, carrot, eggplant, greens, etc., with the exception of potato)
- Grain products (oatmeal, barley, popcorn, brown rice, rye bread, whole-wheat bread, etc.)
- Legumes (peas, beans), nuts, and seeds (almond, pistachio, and sunflower seeds)

Although potato is a vegetable, it is a starch vegetable and low in fiber (only the skin contains dietary fiber).

Foods of animal origin such as meat, poultry, fish, eggs, and dairy products do not contain fiber. Food high in fiber is mostly low in fat, while fatty food has very little fiber.

Soluble versus Insoluble Fiber

Dietary fibers are either soluble or insoluble. Both types are present in all plant food with varying proportions of each:

- Insoluble fiber does not dissolve in water. It has water-attracting properties and helps to increase bulk, soften stool, and shorten the transit time of food through the intestinal tract. Sources of insoluble fiber include whole wheat, wheat and corn bran, and vegetables such as celery, green beans, potato skins, and tomato peel.

- Soluble fiber dissolves in water. It is made of sticky substances like gums, gels, some pectins, and some hemicelluloses. Most soluble fibers can be broken down by the enzymes produced by bacteria in the large intestine, and they undergo metabolic processing via fermentation, which may cause flatus. Because soluble fiber is changed during fermentation, it could provide approximately 2 Calories per gram. Some sources of soluble fiber are legumes (peas, beans), oats, apples, and vegetables (carrots, broccoli, and onions).

Health Benefits of Dietary Fiber

The benefits of dietary fiber include the following:

- Insoluble fiber promotes proper bowel function (preventing constipation). Constipation may cause hemorrhoids or rectal fissures.
- An adequate intake of soluble dietary fiber may cause the following:

  a. Lower cholesterol levels by binding to cholesterol in the gut and increasing its elimination from the body
  b. Lower blood sugar levels and reduced risk of diabetes by attracting water, turning it to gel, and slowing absorption of glucose
  c. Reducing the risk of colorectal cancer by increasing peristalsis and thus limiting the contact of toxins with the lining of the colon or by binding carcinogens

- Dietary fiber may also help to reduce total food intake, because it takes time to chew, and it makes you feel full for a longer time.
- Eating lots of fiber reduces consumption of high-fat and high-calorie food.

How Much Fiber Should People Consume?

The recommended amount of dietary fiber for adolescents and adults is 20–35 g per day, according to the US National Academy of Sciences. A safe range for children is age in years plus 5–10 g per day. For example, a five-year-old child should consume 10–15 g of fiber per day, and fiber intake should approach adult levels (25–30 g) by fifteen years of age.

How Are Americans Doing with Dietary Fiber?

Most American diets are low in fiber, because they are high in fat and low in fruits and vegetables. Foods from animal sources (meat, poultry, fish, eggs, and dairy products) do not have dietary fiber. The average adult gets only around 10 g a day, which is about one-third of the recommended amount (20–35 g). Studies show that only about 5 percent of people eat the recommended amount. In children and adolescents, this value may be as low as 20 percent (Reicks et al. 2014, 226–234).

How to Boost Your Daily Fiber

Emphasizing grains, fresh fruits, and vegetables in your diet will provide adequate fiber (http://www.askdrsears.com/html/4/t041500.asp).

- Consume whole fruits and vegetables instead of juice. The peels on apples and the white pith on oranges are rich sources of fiber, as are potato skins. Don't peel apples and pears. Cut them into easy-to-eat wedges, but leave the skins on.
- Snack on dried fruits such as apricots, figs, prunes, and raisins.

- Consume whole-grain products such as whole-wheat bread, whole-grain cereal, whole-grain cornmeal, wheat germ, barley, and brown rice. White bread and white rice have had the fiber processed out of them.
- Be a bean freak. Nearly all varieties of beans are rich sources of fiber, especially kidney beans, which can be served in salads, soups, burritos, or chili.
- Choose a high-fiber cereal such as bran cereal.
- Choose your lettuce wisely. Iceberg lettuce is useless as a source of fiber and any other nutrients. Spinach and romaine lettuce are healthier choices.
- Fresh fruits have more fiber than canned fruits, because much of the fiber is in the peel, which is usually removed in processing.

The Grain Food Group

Any food made from wheat, rice, corn, or other cereal grains is a grain product. We consume many grain products, including bread, rice, pasta, oatmeal, cereal, and tortillas. The grain group is considered healthy because it provides the body with great sources of energy, dietary fiber, complex carbohydrates, vitamins, and some protein and yet is low in calories. Grain products are divided into whole-grain and refined-grain foods. Most of the health benefits of the grain group come from whole grains; refined-grain products are generally unhealthy.

Whole Grain

A whole grain is the seed of plants like wheat, oats, barley, rye, or rice. A whole grain includes three parts, each with a different store of nutrients (fig. 10.3). Each part has a unique job:

- Endosperm, the core, houses most of the carbohydrate, some protein, and a small amount of vitamins and minerals.
- Bran, the outer layer, contains large amounts of fiber, B vitamins, and minerals.
- Germ contains B vitamins, antioxidants (protecting cells from damage), and phytochemicals. Phytochemicals are naturally produced by plants to protect themselves against viruses, bacteria, and fungi, and they may also enhance immunological defenses.

Examples of whole grains include whole wheat, whole oat, oatmeal, whole-grain corn, popcorn, brown and wild rice, whole rye, whole-grain barley, buckwheat, bulgur (cracked wheat), millet, quinoa, and sorghum.

The health benefits of the grain group are derived from whole-grain products:

- They contain nutrients like folate, B vitamins, and minerals, which are not present in refined grains.
- They are a good source of dietary fiber; refined grain does not have fiber.
- They are a low-GI food. Low-GI food does not produce high levels of blood sugar and insulin and thus may help people prevent becoming overweight or obese.

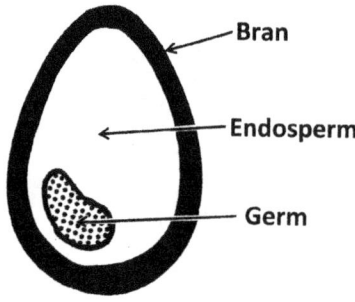

Figure 10.3. Structure of a grain.

Refined Grain

Refined grains are mostly endosperm, because they have been milled, a process that removes bran and germ. This is done to give grains a finer texture and improve their shelf life, but it removes important nutrients such as dietary fiber, iron, and B vitamins.

Examples of refined-grain products are white flour, white bread, and white rice. Most refined grains are enriched. This means that certain B vitamins (thiamin, riboflavin, niacin, folic acid) and iron are added back after processing but fiber is not.

What is the difference between "fortified" and "enriched"?

- Fortified means that nutrients not present in the original food have been added. For example, some varieties of orange juice are fortified with calcium (orange juice normally does not have calcium).
- Enriched means that nutrients originally present in the food have been added back. These are nutrients that may have been lost in processing.

Refined-grain products lose all the health benefits of whole grains. They are high-GI foods that result in unhealthy metabolic effects, and they lack nutrients like dietary fiber, vitamins, and minerals.

How Much Grain Is Recommended Each Day?

The AAP recommends consuming six or more ounces (servings) of grain products per day. Table 10.6 shows the recommended portion size of food groups according to age and gender, which are mostly academic. A simple way of providing enough grain products is to recall MyPlate: a quarter of the plate is filled with the grain food group. Eat as many grain products as you wish, but at least half of them should be whole grains. Consuming more grain products and less meat, fatty food, and sugar-rich food is healthy.

More on "MyPlate"

In the middle of an obesity epidemic, American consumers are bombarded by so many nutrition messages that they are confused about how to improve their diet. Because of that, the food guide pyramid of 1992 and the short-lived MyPyramid of 2005 have been replaced by a simple food plate called MyPlate (fig. 10.4). The older food guide pyramids were criticized for being too complicated for consumers to understand. Built on the 2010 dietary guidelines, MyPlate was released in 2011.

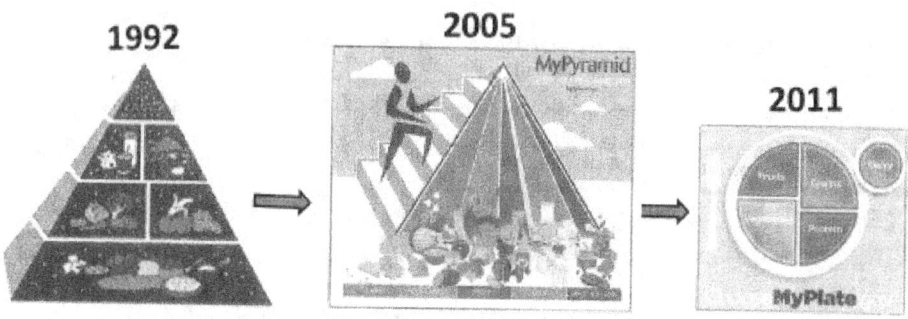

Figure 10.4. Historical changes in food guidance systems recommended by the US government.

MyPlate divides a plate into four labeled sections that show what a balanced meal should look like (fig. 1.4 and fig. 10.4):

- Fruits and vegetables take up half the plate.
- A quadrant on the other side is assigned for grains.
- The last quadrant is assigned for protein.
- Dairy is seen to the side in a circle much like a cup.

The MyPlate icon is easy to understand and consumer friendly, and the dominant message is to consume plant-based foods. Fruits, vegetables, and grains cover three-quarters of the plate. The plate's remaining quadrant is assigned to protein, which may be of animal or plant origin. MyPlate is for everyone who wants to eat healthfully, and it may be especially helpful for people who want to control weight.

For most Americans, it is difficult to eat half a plate of fruits and vegetables every day. It will be difficult for people to eat everyday what MyPlate recommends. The idea here is to eat as closely to MyPlate as possible. MyPlate serves as a constant reminder of how far your diet falls from the ideal. Some people may be concerned that eating this way may cost more or that it will be hard to make healthy choices at restaurants. Both may be true but weight management strategies recommend reducing restaurant food consumption anyway.

Foods That Qualify for Each Food Section

For each section of MyPlate, the foods that qualify are listed below:

- Fruit group. Any fruit or 100 percent fruit juice counts as part of the fruit group. Fruits may be fresh, canned, frozen, or dried.

- Vegetable group. Any vegetable or 100 percent vegetable juice counts as part of the vegetable group. Vegetables may be raw or cooked, fresh, frozen, canned, or dehydrated. Potato is not a healthy choice of vegetable.

- Protein group. It is important to remember that protein may be of animal or plant origin.

  a. Animal sources of protein include meats, poultry, and fish.
  b. Less well-recognized proteins are of plant origin. Dry beans and peas (kidney beans, pinto beans, lima beans, black-eyed peas, and lentils) and soy products such as tofu are examples. These may be counted as vegetables or in the protein food group.

- Grain group. Food made from wheat, rice, oats, cornmeal, barley, or other cereal grains are part of the grain group. Bread, pasta, oatmeal, breakfast cereals, corn, peas, rice, noodles, tortillas, and grits are examples. At least half of the grain products should be whole-grain products.

- Dairy group. All fluid milk products and many foods made from milk are considered part of this group. Fat-free or low-fat varieties are preferred. Foods made from milk that have little or no calcium, such as cream cheese, cream, and butter, do not qualify. Calcium-fortified soy milk (soy beverage) is part of the dairy group.

Fruits and Vegetables

The health benefits of fruits and vegetables are well established, but Americans do not consume enough of them. Although the dietary guideline is five to nine servings of fruits and vegetables a day, according to one national survey the average American eats about three servings of fruits and vegetables a day, and 42 percent eat fewer than two servings a day (Baranowski et al. 1997, 216–223).

The health benefits of fruits and vegetables include the following:

- They are low in calories.
- They are good sources of dietary fiber. Fiber helps regulate bowel movement, lowers blood sugar and cholesterol, and may lower the risk of certain types of cancer.
- Most are excellent sources of vitamins A and C. Vitamin A prevents night blindness, fights infection, and may reduce the risk of certain cancers and heart disease. Vitamin C heals cuts, keeps the skin healthy, and fights infections and colds.
- Eating them makes you feel fuller. They displace high-calorie food and thus help control weight.
- They are high in potassium, which may help to lower blood pressure.

How Much Fruit and Vegetable Food Is Right for My Child?

According to the recommendations of the AHA and the AAP, older children and adolescents should consume 1.5 to 2 cups of fruits and 2.5 to 3 cups of vegetables every day. They should eat 4–5 cups of fruits and vegetables combined every day. Boys need the higher end of the ranges, while girls may need the lower end of the ranges. For more specific information regarding portion size, refer to table 10.6. A simple approach may be to refer to MyPlate, in which half of a plate should be filled with fruits and vegetables. There is no limit to the amount of fruits and vegetables one can take. Although vegetables are generally healthy, some starchy vegetables, like potatoes, should not be consumed in large quantities (see chapter 5).

To encourage Americans to eat more fruits and vegetables, the National Cancer Institute (NCI), with the support of the Produce for Better Health Foundation, started a "Five a Day for Better Health" campaign in 1992. The NCI took it to grocery stores, classrooms, TV, worksites, churches, and elsewhere.

Still another example of encouraging consumption of fruits and vegetables is the 5-2-1-0 message, discussed in chapter 1 (fig. 1.4). The Foundation for Healthy Communities of New Hampshire released the "5-2-1-0 Healthy NH" message in 2006, which was built on the 5-2-1 message developed by Blue Cross Blue Shield of Massachusetts and the 5-2-1-0 campaign used by the Maine Youth Overweight Collaborative. This statewide public education campaign brought awareness to the daily guidelines for nutrition and physical activity. This popular message is simple, clear, and easy to remember, and it represents some of the most important steps families can take to prevent childhood obesity.

The original New Hampshire message was five "servings" a day; it now recommends five "times" a day. "Serving" was used interchangeably with "ounces," because one serving is about one ounce. The old terms "servings" and "ounces" were confusing. According to the old terminology, 1 serving = 1 ounce = ½ cup. It may be better to aim for five cups a day in view of the new serving size recommended by the AHA (see "Recommended Portion Size" in this chapter). The basic message is that there is no limit on the consumption of fruits and vegetables.

Choose Better Vegetables

When considering which vegetables to eat, consider the type of vegetables and the way they are prepared. Not all vegetables are created equal.

- Some vegetables Americans eat are not healthy. According to a report, more than one-third of the total vegetable intake in the United States consists of iceberg lettuce, frozen potatoes (usually French fries), and potato chips. As discussed previously, these are not good choices.

    a. All lettuce, including iceberg and romaine, contains very little fiber and vitamins.
    b. Potatoes, although a vegetable, do not have the nutritional value of leafy vegetables, because they do not contain many vitamins or much fiber and are a high-GI food. The ways potatoes are commonly prepared (such as French fries and potato chips) make them unhealthy. Potatoes and French fries should not be counted as vegetables.
    c. Potato chips should not be counted as vegetables either; they are fatty, salty "junk food."

- Leafy, green, and yellow vegetables are much more nutritious than iceberg lettuce. Examples of healthy vegetables include asparagus, broccoli, celery, Swiss chard, yellow sweet corn, beets, mustard, turnip greens, kale, parsley, snap beans, and spinach.
- Eating a green, leafy salad is good, but too much salad dressing can ruin its healthfulness. Regular salad dressings have large amounts of oil, which is high in calories. Use light or fat-free salad dressing. Measure one tablespoon of dressing, and toss it well with your salad. The dressing coats the salad instead of drenching it.

Energy Density

Energy density, also known as caloric density, refers to the amount of energy (or calories) in a given weight or volume of food. High-energy-density food (or energy-dense food) has a large number of calories relative to its weight or volume, while low-energy-density food has a small number of calories per volume. High-energy-density foods are high in fat and sugar; examples include fried food, butter, bacon, cheese, ice cream, desserts, candies, and soda. Low-energy-density foods have large amounts of water and fiber. Classic examples are fruits, vegetables, and grain products.

In weight control, total calorie intake matters. To reduce the total calorie intake, reduce either the portion size or the energy density of the food.

Research shows that people eat a fairly consistent amount of food on a day-to-day basis. This finding holds true whether the food contains many calories or few calories. People are satisfied only when they take their usual amount of food. Reducing portion size is not an effective strategy. It is difficult for you to ask your overweight child to eat less. You are left with the option of reducing the energy density of the food to decrease calorie intake. Many studies have confirmed that consuming a lower-energy-dense diet can be an effective strategy in weight loss and maintenance (National Center for Chronic Disease Prevention and Health Promotion. 2010). A benefit of this approach is that it allows people to eat satisfying amounts of food while restricting their energy-density intake.

How Is a Low-Energy-Density Food Made?

The factors that play a role in what makes food low in energy density are water and fiber content. Increasing water and fiber content will decrease energy density.

High-fiber food has low calories, but provides volume and takes longer to digest, making you feel full longer on fewer calories. Dietary fiber content is high in fruits, vegetables, and whole-grain products.

High water content in a food makes it a low-energy-density food, because water provides volume but no calories. However, you cannot just add water to food to reduce the calorie density because it would not taste good. Instead, add water-rich vegetables such as zucchini, celery, and carrots to increase water content and reduce calorie density. Increasing fruits, vegetables, and whole-grain products will increase water and fiber contents and result in a low-energy-dense food.

Weight-Control Efforts Using the Concept of Energy Density

Using plenty of fresh fruits, vegetables, and whole grains in preparing meals for the family and reducing portions of high-energy-dense foods are the basis of energy density in weight loss. Make each meal close to MyPlate, in which half of the plate is fruits and vegetables. A few strategies follow, and you can use them alone or in combination:

- Adding blueberries to your cereal in the morning or topping your pasta with sautéed vegetables and tomato sauce are examples of increasing fruit and vegetable portions to reduce energy density.
- You can modify your favorite dish or frequently consumed foods without compromising palatability by adding fruit, vegetables, or grain products or by reducing fat and sugar.
- Incorporate a large portion of fruits and vegetables in your meal plans. Choose spinach, cruciferous vegetables, tomatoes, citrus fruits, and melons for the appetizer, main course, or dessert.
- For your normally high-energy-dense food, you can substitute fat-free or low-fat versions of the ingredients for regular versions.
- For dessert, substitute foods lower in energy density or serve fruits or vegetables.
- Choose meats and cheeses that are lower in fat, or choose poultry or fish.
- Choose water and other low-calorie beverages to quench thirst.

Excessive Salt Intake

Too much sodium can increase your blood pressure and risk of heart attack and stroke. Increased salt consumption in the United States has paralleled the increase in obesity. Americans eat 9–12 g of salt per day or 3,600–4,800 mg of sodium. This is one and a half to two times the recommended amount. Most of it comes from processed foods and restaurant meals, not the saltshaker on the table.

What Is the Daily Sodium Allowance?

In 2005, the US Department of Human Services, the USDA, and the AHA recommended a daily sodium intake of less than 2,300 mg (or 6 g of salt) for adults. The 2010 guidelines recommend 1,500 mg of sodium per day. According to scientific data, the recommended amounts are still more than fifteen to twenty times more the human body requires (He and MacGregor 2010, 363–382). The reduced amount is particularly important information for African Americans, patients with hypertension, and middle-aged and older adults.

The new guidelines recommend increasing consumption of dietary potassium (K), because it helps to attenuate the effect of sodium on blood pressure. Bananas are a well-known source of potassium. Other high-potassium foods include dried apricots, cantaloupe, beets, figs, honeydew melon, orange juice, potatoes (with the skin on), soy products, dairy products, and meats.

Salt versus Sodium

Although we tend to think of the words "salt" and "sodium" as interchangeable, they are not. Table salt is sodium chloride (NaCl), in which 40 percent is sodium and 60 percent is chloride. The amount of salt multiplied by 0.4 gives the amount of sodium, and the amount of sodium multiplied by 2.5 gives the amount of salt (sodium chloride). For example, 2,400 mg of sodium is 6,000 mg (6 g) of salt.

You may have heard of "iodized" or "uniodized" salt. Iodized salt is salt with added iodine. Iodine was added to table salt to prevent a dietary deficiency that caused goiter (swelling of the neck produced by an enlarged thyroid gland). Iodized salt is the most common form of salt. Kosher salt is normally uniodized.

Too much salt intake is unhealthy for the following reasons:

1. High blood pressure. Many studies in diverse populations have shown that high sodium intake is associated with higher blood pressure.
2. Obesity. Increased salt intake is linked to increased obesity. Increasing the intake of sodium, through induction of thirst with increased intake of high-energy beverages, may have contributed to the increase of obesity in the United States.
3. Osteoporosis/bone health. A high salt intake increases the amount of calcium loss in the urine. This increases the risk of osteoporosis and bone fractures. Eating less salt may decrease the loss of calcium from bones.

Health Benefits of Reduced Sodium Intake

Reduced salt intake will achieve the following:

1. Reduce blood pressure levels and decrease the prevalence of obesity.

2. Reduce the incidence of stroke and coronary heart disease, and increase life expectancy.

    (a) A recent thirty-year study from Finland has shown that an average 30–35 percent reduction in salt intake resulted in a dramatic 75–80 percent decrease in stroke and coronary heart disease and increased life expectancy by six to seven years (Vartiainen et al. 1995, 901–904).

    (b) A report from the University of California, San Francisco estimated that every gram of salt reduction would likely result in a quarter of a million fewer deaths (Bibbin-Domingo et al. 2010, 590–599).

How to Reduce Salt Intake

The following suggestions may be useful in reducing your sodium intake. Remember that the most common sources of salt in the United States are processed foods and restaurant meals.

1. At the store

    • Buy fresh or frozen vegetables, fish, shellfish, poultry, and meats. They are lower in salt than most canned and processed forms.

    • Check the nutrition facts label for the sodium content. Generally speaking, foods that are low in sodium contain 140 mg or less per serving (5 percent or less of the daily value per serving).

    • Make it a habit to compare the amount of sodium in processed food when buying high-sodium items like frozen dinners, packaged mixes, cereals, cheese, breads, soups, salad dressings, and sauces.

    • Look for labels that say "low sodium."

2. Cooking and eating at home

    • Make a habit of adding only a small amount of salt when you cook or eat. Learn to use spices and herbs rather than salt to enhance the flavor of food.

    • Leave the saltshaker in a cupboard.

3. Eating out

    • Choose food without sauces like grilled or roasted entrees.

    • Avoid battered and fried food or combination dishes like stews or pasta with sauce. They tend to be high in salt.

    • Ask to have no salt added when the food is prepared.

    • Reduce the frequency of eating restaurant foods.

Good Fat and Bad Fat

When excessive amounts of fats are consumed, they contribute to weight gain, heart disease, and certain types of cancer. However, fats and oils are part of a healthy diet as long as you consume the good kinds of fats. Fats play important roles, such as nerve transmission, maintaining cell membrane integrity, maintaining healthy skin and hair, and maintaining body temperature, by serving as energy stores for the body. They are essential in absorption of fat-soluble vitamins (vitamins A, D, E, and K). The US government and scientific organizations recommend that adults keep their total fat intake to 20–35 percent of calories. Children and adolescents should take 25–35 percent of calories from fats.

In preventing heart disease, the type of the fat is more important than the total amount. Bad fats increase your cholesterol and risk of certain diseases, while good fats have the opposite effect, protecting your heart and supporting overall health. Limit consumption of "bad" fats and consume more "good" fats.

"Good" Fats and "Bad" Fats

Knowing which fats are bad and which fats are good is the first step in lowering the risk of heart disease. Let us consider the four major types of fats: monounsaturated, polyunsaturated, saturated, and trans. Cholesterol is fat bound to a protein.

- "Good" fats are unsaturated (both mono- and polyunsaturated) including omega-3 fatty acids. Unsaturated fats are found mainly in vegetable oils and fish.
- "Bad" fats are saturated and trans fats. Cholesterol in the diet is also a bad fat. Bad fats are found mainly in animal products such as meats and dairy products.

A simple way to identify the types of fat is by appearance. Saturated and trans fats tend to be solid at room temperature (think of the visible fat in meats, butter, or traditional stick margarine). Monounsaturated and polyunsaturated fats tend to be liquid (think of olive or corn oil).

Saturated Fats

- Health effects: Saturated fats raise blood cholesterol, which in turn causes heart disease. They also increase triglyceride levels, which is also a risk factor for heart disease.
- Sources: These include high-fat dairy products, fatty fresh and processed meats, the skin and fat of poultry, lard, palm oil, and coconut oil. Note that tropical plant oils (palm oil, coconut oils) have saturated fats, although most plant oils have unsaturated fats.
- Intake limit: Limit intake to 10 percent of total calories. The 2010 guidelines recommend that only 7 percent of total daily calories come from fat.

- How to reduce saturated fat intake:

  - Eat less red meat (beef, pork, or lamb) and more fish and chicken. Go for lean cuts of meat, and stick to white meat, which has less saturated fat.
  - Remove the skin from chicken, and trim visible fat from meat before cooking.
  - Avoid breaded meats and deep-fried food.
  - Choose low-fat milk and lower-fat cheeses like mozzarella.
  - Use liquid vegetable oils such as olive oil or canola oil instead of lard, shortening, or butter.
  - Avoid cream and cheese sauces, or have them served on the side.
  - Choose healthy alternatives in lieu of saturated fats (see box 10.1).

Box 10.1 Sources of saturated fats and their healthier options

SOURCES OF SATURATED FATS	HEALTHIER OPTIONS
Butter	Olive oil
Cheese	Low-fat or reduced-fat cheese
Red meat	White-meat chicken or turkey
Cream	Low-fat milk or fat-free creamer
Eggs	Egg whites, an egg substitute (e.g., Eggbeaters), or tofu
Ice cream	Frozen yogurt or reduced-fat ice cream
Whole milk	Skim or 1% milk
Sour cream	Plain, nonfat yogurt

Trans Fatty Acids

Trans fatty acids are artificial saturated fats produced from unsaturated fatty acids by a process called hydrogenation (the addition of hydrogen). The process turns liquid oils, such as corn oil, into solid fat that can be used in products.

- Health effects: Trans fats act like saturated fats, raising cholesterol levels and clogging coronary arteries. Compared to saturated fat, trans fatty acids are associated with a 2.5–10 times greater risk of heart disease. Like saturated fats, trans fats also increase triglyceride levels.

- Sources: The primary source of trans fat in the American diet is commercially prepared baked goods and snack food (40 percent), such as cakes, cookies, crackers, pies, and bread. Other sources of trans fat include animal products (21 percent), margarine (17 percent), French fries (8 percent), and chips and popcorn (5 percent). Box 10.2 lists common sources of trans fats.

- Intake limit: There is no daily allowance for trans fat, but it should be limited as much as possible. Note that trans fat levels of less than 0.5 g per serving can be listed as 0 gram trans fat on the food label.

- How to reduce trans fat intake:

  - When shopping, check the food label for trans fats.
  - When eating out, avoid fried food, biscuits, and other baked goods, unless you know that the restaurant has eliminated trans fat.
  - Avoid fast food.
  - When cooking, avoid using cooking oils that are high in saturated fats and/or trans fats such as coconut oil, palm oil, or vegetable shortening. Use canola, olive, and flax seed oil instead.
  - Minimize eating commercially packaged foods that are high in trans fats such as cakes, cookies, crackers, and pies.

Box 10.2 Common sources of trans fats

CATEGORY	EXAMPLES
Baked goods	Cookies, crackers, cakes, muffins, pie crusts, pizza dough, and some breads like hamburger buns
Fried food	Donuts, French fries, fried chicken, chicken nuggets, and hard taco shells
Snack food	Potato, corn, and tortilla chips; candy; packaged or microwave popcorn
Solid fats	Stick margarine and semisolid vegetable shortening
Premixed products	Cake mix, pancake mix, and chocolate drink mix

- State and Local Regulation in the United States. The state of California and some US cities are acting to reduce consumption of trans fats. In May 2005, Tiburon, California, became the first American city where all restaurants voluntarily cook with trans fat–free oils. Since then, many other cities and counties have passed laws to help reduce the amount of trans fats in restaurants. Included in the list are New York, Philadelphia, San Francisco, Montgomery County (Maryland), Nassau County (New York), and Albany County (New York). California became the first state to ban trans fats in restaurants, effective January 1, 2010, but packaged foods are not covered by the ban and can still legally contain trans fats.

Dietary Cholesterol

- Health effects: There is a great misunderstanding about cholesterol on food labels. Part of the confusion comes from the fact that cholesterol in food is not the same thing as the serum cholesterol, which clogs arteries. Foods high in cholesterol can cause cholesterol to rise but only rarely. Dietary cholesterol is only about half as important as saturated and trans fat in raising serum cholesterol levels. The biggest influence on serum cholesterol is the bad fats (saturated fat and trans fat). Cholesterol in one's diet is far less important. Instead of counting the cholesterol in food, focus on saturated and trans fats.

Some foods are labeled as being "cholesterol-free" or "low in cholesterol." This does not mean much, because some foods loaded with saturated or trans fats can be labeled as containing zero cholesterol, but they are more of a threat to your heart than foods with a little cholesterol and less saturated fat.

- Sources: Foods such as egg yolks, meat, and dairy fats are high in cholesterol, but they contribute little to high serum LDL cholesterol. Plant foods such as fruits, vegetables, and grain products do not contain cholesterol.
- Intake limit: Limit cholesterol intake to 300 mg per day. The 2010 dietary guidelines recommend reducing it to 200 mg in persons at risk for heart disease and type 2 diabetes.

How About an Egg?

Many adults eat eggs at breakfast. This is the nutritional content of a large egg:
- The whole egg provides 71 Calories, while the egg white provides 17 Calories. The whole egg is mostly protein with some fat and cholesterol in the egg yolk. There is no carbohydrate.
- Egg yolk contains 5 g of fat and 211 mg of cholesterol. The egg white has no fat or cholesterol.

Cholesterol in a large egg accounts for two-thirds of the recommended daily limit. Researchers indicate that cholesterol in food is not the culprit. Saturated fat from other food (dairy products, fatty meats) has a much bigger effect on blood cholesterol (Kritchevsky 2004,596S–600S).

According to the AHA, there is no reason that whole eggs can't be part of a heart-healthy diet in adults. It's fine to eat one whole egg a day as long as the rest of the day a person follows a low-cholesterol diet. For those with heart conditions, high cholesterol, or any risk factors for heart disease, it is best to cut back on egg yolk consumption or use egg whites only. For children, eating an occasional egg should pose no health risk.

Unsaturated Fats

- Health effects: Unsaturated fats and oils do not raise blood cholesterol and are healthy fats, although excess amounts will cause weight gain.
- Sources: Unsaturated fats occur in vegetable oils, most nuts, olives, avocados, and fatty fish like salmon. Unsaturated oils include monounsaturated fats and polyunsaturated fats.
  a. Monounsaturated fatty acids come from plants. Monounsaturated fats are liquid at room temperature, and they get thicker when chilled. Examples of monounsaturated fats include olive oil, canola oil, sunflower oil, peanut oil, sesame oil, avocados, olives, nuts (almonds, peanuts, macadamia nuts, hazelnuts, pecans, cashews), and peanut butter.

b. Polyunsaturated fats include plants and fish. Polyunsaturated fats are liquid at room temperature, and they stay liquid when chilled. Plant sources of polyunsaturated fatty acids include soybean oil, corn oil, safflower oil, cottonseed oil, walnuts, sunflower, sesame, pumpkin seeds, flaxseed, soy milk, and tofu. Omega-3 fatty acids come from fish sources of polyunsaturated fatty acids (salmon, tuna, mackerel, herring, trout, and sardines).

- Intake limit: It is recommended that 20–35 percent of calories should come from sources of polyunsaturated and monounsaturated fatty acids.

Omega-3 Fatty Acids

Omega-3 fatty acids belong to polyunsaturated fatty acids. Omega-3 fats are a type of essential fatty acid, meaning that your body can't make them. They are essential to health, so you need to take them.

There are different types of omega-3 fatty acids:

a. Eicosapentaenoic acid (EPA) and docosahexaenoic acid (DHA) are found in abundance in cold-water, fatty fish.
b. Alpha-linolenic acid (ALA) comes from plants. It is a less potent form of omega-3 than EPA and DHA. The best sources include flaxseed, walnuts, and canola oil.

- Health effects: Omega-3 fatty acids provide health benefits in both physical and mental health. They play a vital role in cognitive function (memory, problem-solving abilities, etc.) and emotional health. They help prevent heart disease and stroke. They may lower triglycerides and LDL cholesterol and increase good HDL cholesterol.
- Sources: The best sources of omega-3 fatty acids are fatty fish such as salmon, herring, mackerel, anchovies, or sardines, or high-quality cold-water fish oil supplements. Canned albacore tuna and lake trout can also be good sources.
- Intake limit: Some people avoid seafood, because they worry about mercury or other possible toxins. However, most experts agree that the benefits of eating two servings a week of cold-water, fatty fish outweigh the risks.

How to Reduce Fat Intake

Most American foods are high in fat, and eating too much of high-fat food may have contributed to your child's weight problem. Reducing fat intake is an excellent way to cut down overall calories and thus control weight. Fat accounts for more than two times the calories than those provided by carbohydrate and protein in food. Remember that 1 g of fat equals 9 Calories, while 1 g of protein or carbohydrate equals 4 Calories.

Strategies to Reduce Fat Intake

Whether you are trying to lose weight, lower blood cholesterol, or eat healthier, you'll want to limit total fat intake. This effort should be in parallel with efforts to make up for the reduced amount of fat; simply attempting to reduce fat intake will not succeed. The actions you need to take are as follows:

- Eat plenty of low-fat, plant-based foods (whole grains, fruits, and vegetables) that give you satisfying portions but are low in calories.
- Limit your meat consumption to less than 6 oz. per day.
- Choose only reduced-fat or fat-free dairy products (table 10.5).
- Use plant protein, such as in beans and lentils, which is a low-fat, cholesterol-free protein, at meals or snacks in place of animal protein.
- Increase your physical activity to improve heart health and lose excess body fat.

How to Reduce Fat Intake

There are three ways to reduce fat intake:

1. Smart grocery shopping
   - Food labels help you determine how much fat is in the food. Learn how to read the food label (described in chapter 5). Choose food low in fat by checking the percent DV. An amount greater than 20 percent of percent DV is considered high; one less than 5 percent is considered low.
   - Choose lean meats, fish, and poultry. Limit these to less than 6 oz. per day.
   - Other low-fat sources of protein include dried beans and peas, tofu, low-fat yogurt, low-fat milk, low-fat cottage cheese, and tuna fish packed in water (see table 10.7)
   - Choose skim or 1 percent milk.
   - Choose reduced- or low-fat dairy products, including low-fat cheeses (no more than 3 g of fat per oz.) or nonfat cheeses or spreads (see table 10.5).
   - Try low-fat or fat-free versions of your favorite margarine, salad dressing, cream cheese, and mayonnaise.
   - Buy low-fat snacks. Avoid chips (potato, corn, and others) that are high in fat and salt.
   - Buy fruits, vegetables, and grain products in lieu of meat and dairy products.

- Buy fewer processed foods. Buy products in their natural state, and cook them at home in a healthful way. Processing often strips food of fiber, vitamins, and minerals while adding fat, sugar, salt, and chemicals.
- Refer to table 10.5, which provides lists of high-fat foods and their low-fat alternative for dairy products, meat, fish, poultry, and other grocery items.

2. Healthy food preparation

Even if you have shopped in a healthy way, unhealthy cooking methods can add fats to your food. The following lists some healthy cooking methods:

- Trim fat from meats, and remove skin from poultry before cooking.
- Bake, grill, or broil, and avoid deep-frying or pan-frying. Stir-frying or sautéing is a better way to cook with oil.
- Use nonstick vegetable oil cooking spray instead of liquid oil.
- Use olive and canola oils for all cooking and baking needs.
- If a recipe calls for butter or lard, substitute olive or canola oil.
- When the recipe calls for cheese, use half the amount called for, or substitute reduced-fat cheeses.
- Refrigerate soups, gravies, and stews, and remove the hardened fat before eating.
- Replace meat dishes with fish, beans, or tofu (which provide good-quality protein but a small amount of fat).

3. Healthy eating behaviors

- Reduce the frequency of eating out and takeout food. Restaurant food is in general high in fat and salt, and eating out usually results in overeating.
- When you have to eat fast food, it is still possible to make nutritious selections:

  - Order a grilled or charbroiled chicken sandwich without skin and mayonnaise, and do the fixing "your way."
  - Order a lean roast beef sandwich.
  - Keep the portions to regular and small (no "double" anything or "going large").
  - Order food without the cheese.
  - Request that your food be cooked without added butter, margarine, gravy, or sauces.
  - Order skim or 1 percent milk rather than a high-fat shake (or high-sugar soda). Water is the best drink.
  - Order a salad with a small amount of low-fat dressing.
  - Select fruits, angel food cake, nonfat frozen yogurt, sherbet, or sorbet for dessert instead of ice cream, cake, or pie.

Table 10.5 Low-calorie, lower-fat alternative foods

HIGHER-FAT FOODS	LOWER-FAT FOODS
DAIRY PRODUCTS	
Evaporated whole milk	Evaporated fat-free (skim) or reduced-fat (2 %) milk
Whole milk	Low-fat (1 %), reduced-fat (2 %), or fat-free (skim) milk
Ice cream	Sorbet, sherbet, low-fat or fat-free frozen yogurt, or ice
Whipping creams	Imitation whipped cream (made with fat-free [skim] milk)
Sour cream	Plain low-fat yogurt
Cream cheese	Neufchatel or "light" cream cheese or fat-free cream cheese
Cheese (cheddar, Swiss, and jack)	Reduced-calorie cheese, low-calorie processed cheeses, etc. Fat-free cheese
American cheese	Fat-free American cheese or other types of fat-free cheeses
Regular (4 %) cottage cheese	Low-fat (1 %) or reduced-fat (2 %) cottage cheese
Whole milk mozzarella cheese	Part-skim milk, low-moisture mozzarella cheese
Whole milk ricotta cheese	Part-skim milk ricotta cheese
Coffee cream (1/2 and ½) or nondairy creamer (liquid, powder)	Low-fat (1 %) or reduced-fat (2%) milk or nonfat dry milk powder
MEAT, FISH, AND POULTRY	
Cold-cuts or lunch meats (bologna, salami, liverwurst, etc.)	Low-fat cold cuts (95–97 %), fat-free lunch meats, low-fat lunch meats, and low-fat pressed meats
Hot dogs (regular)	Lower-fat hot dogs
Bacon or sausage	Canadian bacon or lean ham
Regular ground beef	Extra-lean ground beef such as ground round or ground turkey (read label)
Chicken or turkey with skin, duck, or goose	Chicken or turkey without skin (white meat)
Oil-packed tuna	Water-packed tuna (rinse to reduce sodium content)
Beef (chuck rib, brisket)	Beef (round, loin) (trimmed of external fat) (choose select grade)
Pork (spareribs, untrimmed loin)	Pork tenderloin or trimmed, lean smoked ham
Frozen breaded fish or fried fish (homemade or commercial)	Fish or shellfish, unbreaded (fresh, frozen, canned in water)
Whole eggs	Egg whites or egg substitutes
Frozen TV dinners (containing more than 13 g of fat per serving)	Frozen TV dinners (containing less than 13 g. of fat per serving and lower in sodium)
Chorizo sausage	Turkey sausage, drained well (read label) Vegetarian sausage (made with tofu)

Table 10.5 Low-calorie, lower-fat alternative foods (Continued.)

HIGHER-FAT FOODS	LOWER-FAT FOODS
CEREALS, GRAINS, AND PASTAS	
Ramen noodles	Rice or noodles (spaghetti, macaroni, etc.)
Pasta with white sauce (Alfredo)	Pasta with red sauce (marinara)
Pasta with cheese sauce	Pasta with vegetables (primavera)
Granola	Bran flakes, crispy rice, etc. Cooked grits or oatmeal Reduced-fat granola
BAKED GOODS	
Croissants, brioches, etc.	Hard French rolls or soft brown 'n serve rolls
Donuts, sweet rolls, muffins, scones, or pastries	English muffins, bagels, reduced-fat or fat-free muffins or scones (choose lowest calorie variety)
Party crackers	Low-fat crackers (choose lowest in sodium) Saltine or soda crackers (choose lowest in sodium)
Cake (pound, chocolate, yellow)	Cake (angel food, white, and gingerbread)
Cookies	Reduced-fat or fat-free cookies (graham crackers, ginger snaps, and fig bars)(choose lowest calorie variety)
SNACKS AND SWEETS	
Nuts	Popcorn (air-popped or light microwave), fruits, vegetables
Ice cream, e.g., cones or bars	Frozen yogurt, frozen fruit, or chocolate pudding bars
Custards or puddings (made with whole milk)	Puddings (made with skim milk)
FATS, OILS, AND SALAD DRESSINGS	
Regular margarine or butter	Light spread margarines, diet margarine, or whipped butter, tub or squeeze bottle
Regular mayonnaise	Light or diet mayonnaise or mustard
Regular salad dressings	Reduced-calorie or fat-free salad dressings, lemon juice, or plain, herb flavored, or wine vinegar
Butter or margarine on toast or bread	Jelly, jam, or honey on bread or toast
Oils, shortening, or lard	Nonstick cooking spray for stir-frying or sautéing As a substitute for oil or butter, use applesauce or prune puree in baked goods
MISCELLANEOUS	
Canned cream soups	Canned broth-based soups
Canned beans and franks	Canned baked beans in tomato sauce
Gravy (homemade with fat and/or milk)	Gravy mixes made with water or homemade with the fat skimmed off and fat-free milk
Fudge sauce	Chocolate syrup
Avocado on sandwiches	Cucumber slices or lettuce leaves
Guacamole dip or refried beans with lard	Salsa

Modified from National Heart, Lung and Blood Institute, "Low-calorie, low fat alternative foods." http://www.nhlbi.nih.gov/health/educational/lose_wt/eat/shop_lcal_fat.htm.

Energy Drinks and Sports Drinks

Energy Drinks

So-called "energy drinks" are advertised as providing energy to improve physical activity. A variety of brands are available: Red Bull, Cocaine, SoBe Adrenaline Rush, Tab Energy, Snapple Fire, Blue Ox, Power House, and Atomic Energy. The advertisers claim increased energy, metabolism, stamina, and mental alertness.

The central ingredient in most energy drinks is caffeine, the same stimulant found in coffee or tea. Energy drinks may contain other stimulants like guarana (a South African plant that supplies a caffeine-like substance), ginseng, acai, taurine, various amino acids, vitamins, minerals, and herbs. Caffeine is a well-known stimulant of the central nervous system, so energy drinks can induce mild to moderate euphoria and improve physical activity by increasing muscle endurance. However, the effects last for a short time and then drop off, just like drinking a cup of coffee.

Compare the amount of caffeine in energy drinks to 100 mg of caffeine in a cup of coffee:

- AMP, 74 mg (8.4 oz.)
- Enviga, 100 mg (12 oz.)
- Full Throttle, 144 mg (16 oz.)
- Jolt, 71.2 mg (12 oz.)
- Monster Energy, 160 mg (12 oz.)
- No Fear, 83 mg (8 oz.)
- No Name (formerly known as "Cocaine"), 280 mg (8.4 oz.)
- Red Bull, 80 mg (8.4 oz.)
- SoBe Adrenaline Rush, 78 mg (8.45 oz.)
- Tab Energy, 72 mg (8 oz.)

There are side effects and potential dangers if energy drinks are consumed excessively. Side effects may include agitation, anxiety, insomnia, nausea, vomiting, heart rhythm irregularities, and high blood pressure. These side effects are of particular concern in children. How quickly the drink is consumed can result in more serious side effects. People usually drink coffee slowly, but energy drinks are often consumed rapidly to quench thirst during or after physical activities. Some people may drink more than one container of an energy drink, thinking that it may increase physical performance proportionally. Among pregnant women, high caffeine intake is associated with the risk of miscarriage, stillbirth, and infants who are small for their gestational age. At least one death has been reported among young athletes consuming energy drinks. Because of these concerns, energy drinks have been banned in some countries (like France).

Other Food and Drinks with Caffeine

Besides energy drinks, other drinks and food that children consume have caffeine. Consumption of too much food with caffeine can cause a fast heart rate and a rise in blood pressure, and it may disrupt normal sleep patterns. The AAP recommends that adolescents consume no more than 100 mg of caffeine a day. Smaller children should consume less than this amount.

The following is a general guide to the amount of caffeine in various foods. One can easily compare it to the amount of caffeine in a cup of coffee:

- The caffeine in an average cup of coffee (8 oz.) is 80–150 mg, averaging 100 mg.
- Decaffeinated coffee (8 oz.) has 5–10 mg of caffeine.
- Teas (8 oz.) have 40–50 mg of caffeine, although this varies widely by type and brand. Black tea has a higher amount of caffeine than green tea.
- The caffeine content in energy drinks ranges from 80–280 mg per container, which may come in 8 oz. or 16 oz. sizes.
- Most soft drinks (12 oz.) contain about 40 mg of caffeine. For example, A&W Cream Soda, Dr. Pepper, and Diet Dr. Pepper have a little less, and Pepsi Max and Diet Pepsi Max have a little more.
- Soft drinks such as 7-Up, Sprite, Fresca, Fanta, Slice, Sierra Mist, and Mug Root Beer do not have caffeine.
- There is caffeine in chocolate but only small amounts. Dark chocolate has 20 mg in 1 oz., milk chocolate has 6 mg in 1 oz., white chocolate has 0 mg in 1 oz., and chocolate milk has 4 mg in 8 oz.

Sports Drinks

Sports drinks should not be confused with energy drinks. Energy drinks are highly caffeinated and may contain other stimulants, while sports drinks do not contain caffeine. Sports drinks such as Gatorade, Powerade, and Allsport are formulated to supply optimal amounts of carbohydrates and electrolytes for endurance, rehydrating, and balancing body chemistry after physical activity. However, excessive consumption of sports drinks may cause excess calorie intake. Gatorade has 13 gm of sugar in 8 oz. compared to Coca-Cola, which has about 27 gm of sugar in the same volume. Gatorade 2 is a low-calorie version that has 7 gm of sugar in 8 oz.

If the exercise lasts less than one hour, drink plain water. For extended periods of exercise (more than one hour), sports drinks containing carbohydrates and electrolytes help prevent dehydration and restore important minerals lost through perspiration.

Recommended Portion Size

A healthy diet requires reduced consumption of certain food groups and increased consumption of others. The former includes added sugars, solid fat, refined grains, and sodium, and the latter includes fruits, vegetables, whole-grain products, low-fat milk, and seafood. MyPlate emphasizes the importance of fruits, vegetables, and grain products. In addition, the dietary guidelines for Americans emphasize reducing the consumption of SoFAS. As long as your serving plate is close to MyPlate and you reduce SoFAS, it is not important to know the exact recommended portion of each food group, but this information may be useful under certain circumstances.

What Is the Appropriate Portion Size?

The amount of food a child needs depends on the child's age, whether the child is a girl or a boy, and how active the child is. Although small children may need smaller amounts of food than older children, they still need the same variety of food as adults.

Table 10.6 shows the recommended servings for the food groups according to calorie needs, shown by age and gender. These AHA guidelines were endorsed by the AAP in 2006. The recommended servings are similar to table 10.6. Note that the table is based on a sedentary lifestyle. Children who are more active burn more calories, so they need more food. Moderately active persons may require an additional 200 kcal per day (200–400 kcal per day for very active individuals). Accordingly, the portion size needs to be adjusted.

Table 10.6 Daily estimated calories and recommended servings for grains, fruits, vegetables, and milk/dairy*

	GIRLS			BOYS		
	4–8 yr.	9–13 yr.	14–18 yr.	4–8 yr.	9–13 yr.	14–18 yr.
Kilocalories	1,200	1,600	1,800	1400	1,800	2,200
Fat (% total kcal)		25–35%			25–35%	
Milk/dairy (cups)	2	3	3	2	3	3
Lean meat/beans (oz.)	3	5	5	4	5	6
Fruits (cups)	1.5	1.5	1.5	1.5	1.5	2
Vegetables (cups)	1	2	2.5	1.5	2.5	3
Grains (oz.)	4	5	6	5	6	7

* Based on sedentary lifestyle.
Adapted from S. S. Gidding et al., "Dietary Recommendations for Children and Adolescents: A Guide for Practitioners." *Pediatrics* 117 (2006): 544–559.

Recommended Serving Size

Recommendations by the US government used "servings" to express the amount of food, as found on the old food pyramid, but "serving" is a confusing term. "One serving" is an arbitrary unit, and most people are not familiar with the unit. It needs to be converted to common household measures like "cup" to make sense. The new recommendations by the AHA are more user-friendly and appear in household measures like cups and ounces. Remember that one serving is about 1 oz., and 1 oz. is about ½ cup.

In table 10.6, fruits and vegetables are expressed in cups, but grains and meats are expressed in ounces. It is not easy to know how much 1 oz. of bread, cereal, meat, or fish is. The following will help.

For the grain group, each of the following equals about 1 oz.:

> 1 slice of bread or dinner roll
> 1 tortilla (6-inch diameter)
> 1 pancake or waffle (4-inch diameter)
> ½ English muffin, hamburger roll, pita, or bagel (frozen; those from bagel shops can be up to four servings)
> ½ cup of cooked rice, pasta, or barley
> ½ cup of cooked oatmeal, grits, or Cream of Wheat cereal
> 1 cup of cold cereal
> Three to four small crackers

For the meat, fish, and bean group, each of the following equals about 1 oz.:

> ¼ cup cooked dry beans
> 1 egg
> 1 tablespoon of peanut butter
> A deck of standard 52 playing cards equals 3 oz. of meat, poultry, or fish
> A small handful of nuts or seeds

What Is the Difference Between Serving Size and Portion Size?

Some articles, books, and websites use the terms "serving size" and "portion size" interchangeably, but they are not interchangeable. A *serving size* (used in the nutrition facts label and in the old food pyramid) is a unit of measure that was determined by the USDA and based on nationwide food consumption surveys. This is the amount of the food usually eaten at one time. A *portion size* is the amount of a food that you *choose* to eat. You could be eating twice more or half of the serving size, but either one is your portion size.

Fish and Seafood

Eating seafood allows for a greater variety of food in your diet. Seafood is readily available and relatively inexpensive, and it provides nutritious protein and beneficial fat, which contribute to a healthful diet.

Nutritional Facts of Seafood

Fish is in general healthier than red meat because of the following:

- It is an excellent source of high-quality protein (like a red meat).
- It is lower in saturated fat and calories than beef or pork.
- It contains an abundance of omega-3 fatty acids, which are not found in red meat.
- It is loaded with B vitamins and minerals such as iron, zinc, and calcium (found in canned fish with soft, edible bones).

Health Benefits of Omega-3 Fatty Acids

The health benefits of fish come primarily from omega-3s, which are polyunsaturated fatty acids. Two important omega-3s are EPA and DHA. Omega-3s are essential fatty acids, meaning they cannot be synthesized in the body and must be obtained from food. Evidence continues to build, revealing how seafood omega-3s may improve health.

These are the health benefits of omega-3s:

- Heart Health. Helps lower triglycerides and increase HDL cholesterol, thereby lowering the risk of heart disease

  a. Lowers blood pressure
  b. Acts as an anticoagulant to prevent blood clots, reducing the incidence of stroke
  c. Improves electrical properties of the heart, including more stable rhythm and reduced chance of irregular rhythm

- Brain Function. It supports proper brain growth and development in fetal and infant life; insufficient intake of omega-3s is associated with a greater chance of childhood behavioral disorders such as dyslexia, ADHD, and conditions affecting movement and coordination. It may protect against Alzheimer's disease and other dementias and Parkinson's disease
- Mental Health. It reduces the risk and severity of several mental disorders, including depression, bipolar disorder, and mood disorders such as anxiety, hostility, and aggression
- Visual Function. It may lower the chance of developing age-related macular degeneration and possibly cataract, dry eye, glaucoma, and other visual disorders. It promotes healthy visual development in early infancy
- Immune Function. Promotes immune system maturation in infancy and may lower the chance of childhood allergies

- Healthy Pregnancy. Needed for infant brain and eye development, brain structure and function, and visual acuity

Sources of Omega-3 Fatty Acids

Omega-3 fatty acids are found throughout the aquatic food chain, and all fish and shellfish used for human food are sources. Although not all fish are high in omega-3 fatty acids, they still can contribute important amounts of fatty acids if eaten regularly.

In general, the amount of omega-3 fatty acids is related to the total fat content of the species:

- Darker fleshed, oily fish such as herring, salmon, mackerel, and bluefish generally have a higher total fat and omega-3 content.
- Leaner fish with lighter-colored flesh such as cod, flounder, and pollack have lower amounts of fat and omega-3 content.

Table 10.7 shows the omega-3 fatty acid content of some of the most frequently consumed fish and shellfish species in the United States.

Table 10.7 Omega-3 content of frequently consumed seafood products

OMEGA-3 PER 3 OZ. COOKED PORTION	SEAFOOD PRODUCT
> 1,500 mg	Herring (W), salmon (F & W), mackerel (W)
1,000–1,500 mg	Salmon (C), Mackerel (C & W), tuna (W)
500–1,000 mg	Salmon (W), sardines (C), tuna (C), swordfish (W), trout (F), oysters (W & F), mussels (F & W)
200–500 mg	Tuna (C), tuna (W), pollock (W), rockfish (W), clams (F & W), crab (W), lobster (W), snapper (W), grouper (W), flounder/sole (W), halibut (W), ocean perch (W), squid (W), fish sticks (B)
< 200 mg	Scallops (W), shrimp (W & F), lobster (W), crab (W), cod (W), haddock (W), tilapia (F), catfish (F), mahimahi (W), tuna (W), orange roughy (W), surimi product (imitation crab)

W = Wild; F = Farmed; C = Canned; B = Breaded.
Source: USDA National Nutrient Database for Standard Reference., "Seafood & Nutrition: General Information for Healthcare Professionals."
[http://seafoodhealthfacts.org/seafood_nutrition/practitioners/omega3_content.php]

How Much Fish Is Recommended?

Compared with meat and poultry, Americans eat little seafood (about ½ oz. a day versus 7½ oz. a day for meat and poultry).

US health organizations recommend consuming at least 250–500 mg of omega-3 fatty acids per day or at least two servings per week of oily fish.

Experts from the Food and Agriculture Organization (FAO) of the United Nations and the WHO recommend that DHA should account for at least 200 mg of the daily intake for pregnant or nursing women, and the daily EPA + DHA intake among children should be 100–250 mg.

The AHA recommends 1,000 mg omega-3 fatty acids per day for patients with coronary heart disease.

The 2010 dietary guidelines for Americans advise eating a variety of seafood twice per week (8 oz. or more), which will provide the recommended 250 mg per day for optimal health. Only one in five Americans currently meets the guideline.

Seafood Safety Issues

Despite the demonstrated positive health effects of seafood, there are potential hazards. Many people have raised questions about the trace levels of contaminants such as mercury and polychlorinated biphenyls (PCB) found in fish. However, researchers at the Harvard Center for Risk Analysis concluded that the risks of not eating fish are greater than any risks associated with eating fish (Willett 2005, 320–321).

1. Mercury in fish
    Nearly all fish and shellfish contain traces of mercury. For most people, the risk from mercury by eating fish and shellfish is not a health concern. However, some fish and shellfish that contain higher levels of mercury may be harmful to pregnant women, infants, and children because they may harm the developing nervous system. Methylmercury is the toxic form. The US government advises that women who may become pregnant, pregnant women, nursing mothers, and young children avoid some types of fish and eat fish and shellfish that are lower in mercury.

    *   Do not eat large predatory fish such as shark, swordfish, king mackerel, or tilefish because they contain high levels of mercury.
    *   Five of the most commonly eaten fish that are low in mercury are shrimp, canned light tuna, salmon, Pollock, and catfish.

2. PBCs in farm-raised salmon
    Although salmon provides healthful nutrients, farm-raised salmon present health concerns:

    *   Farmed salmon are contaminated with PCBs at levels that raise health concerns (according to laboratory tests commissioned by the Environmental Working Group) (Environmental Working Group 2003). Farmed salmon in US grocery stores are likely the most PCB-contaminated protein source in the US food supply. On average, farmed salmon have sixteen times the dioxin-like PCBs

found in wild salmon, four times the levels found in beef, and 3.4 times the levels found in other seafood. Dried food pellets for farm-raised salmons are often contaminated with cancer-causing agents as PCBs, dioxins, and even flame retardants.

- Because they are raised in crowded living conditions, farm-raised salmon are given antibiotics to prevent infection. Some sources say that salmon are given more antibiotics than any other form of livestock (Green Philly 2013).

- Farm-raised salmon have far lower levels of omega-3 fatty acids than their wild counterparts. They also have higher levels of omega-6 fatty acids (a pro-inflammatory type of fatty acid).

Detailed Nutrition Facts

The Nutrition Labeling and Education Acts went into effect in 1990 to help the public to eat food that does not have excessive calories, fat, sugar, and sodium and adequate amounts of nutrients, vitamins, minerals, and dietary fiber.

You learned in chapter 5 how to check the food label to reduce fat and sugar intake and help control weight. By now you may feel comfortable with the notations for serving size, calories per serving, percent DV of fat, and amount of sugar. The next level would be to know the following:

- More in-depth information about the above four elements
- How to limit intake of sodium and cholesterol
- How to increase intake of dietary fiber and vitamins
- What else can be learned from the food label?

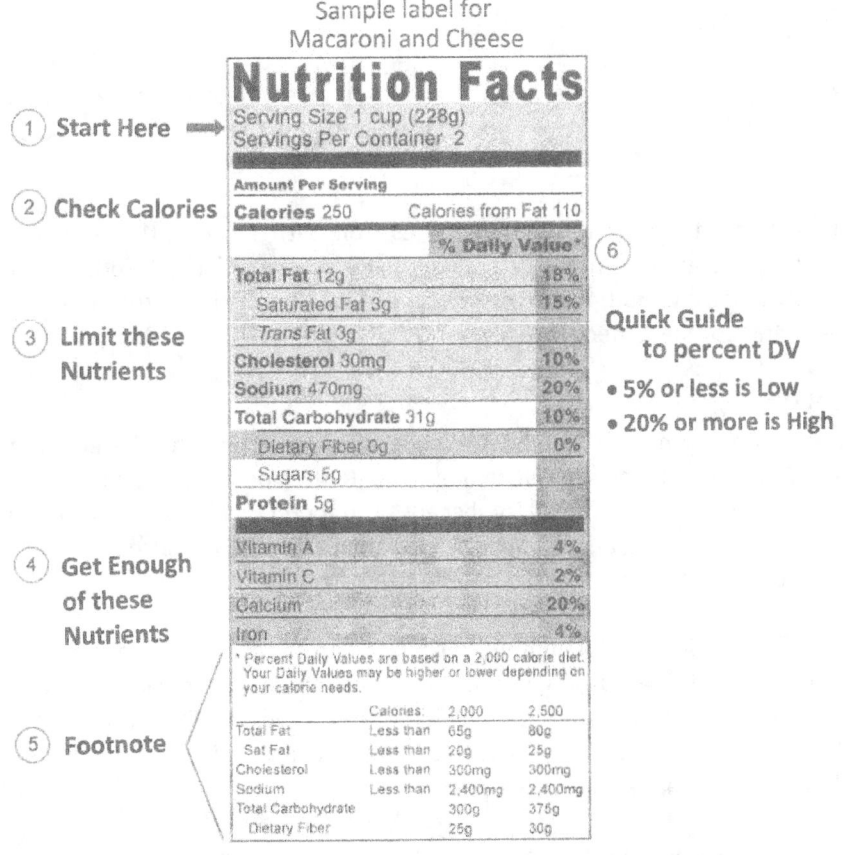

Figure 10.5. Nutrition facts of packaged macaroni and cheese.

1. Serving Size

The first place to start is the serving size and the number of servings in the package. All the nutrient values shown on the label are based on *one serving* of the food. Pay attention to the serving size and the number of servings you are going to eat (portion size). For example, if you decide to eat two servings, double the calories and other nutrient numbers, including the percent DV. If you decide to eat two cups of macaroni and cheese (fig. 10.5), your total fat percent DV increases to 36 percent, which is high.

2. Calories

Calories provide a measure of how much energy you get from a serving of food. The number of servings you consume determines the number of calories you actually eat. In general, the calorie number in a serving gives you a good idea about calorie density of the food.

- 40 Calories is low
- 100 Calories is moderate
- 400 Calories or more is high

As shown in fig. 10.5, there are 250 Calories in one serving of macaroni and cheese, which is moderate. If you eat two cups of macaroni and cheese, you eat 500 Calories, which is high.

It is not necessary to check the item "calories from fat," because this number will be determined by the amount of fat in a serving. The number of 110 Calories in this case can be determined by multiplying the grams of fat (12 g in this case) by 9. If you are interested in fat content, check the percent DV of total fat.

3. Percent DV

The percent DV is a convenient number to check when shopping. It is based on the daily value recommendations for key nutrients for a 2,000-Calorie diet. You do not need to know how to calculate the percent DV, because the food label has done the calculation. The percent DV does not add up to 100 percent vertically, because each nutrient is based on 100 percent of the daily requirement for that nutrient.

The percent DV is also a useful number to check when shopping. It helps you determine if a serving of food is high or low in a nutrient. You can also compare similar foods to determine which food is higher in nutrients and lower in fats. When comparing products, consider the serving sizes, because they may differ. It is important to remember the following regarding the percent DV:

- Five percent or less is low.
- Twenty percent or more is high.

These numbers are useful for *all* nutrients: those you want to limit (fat, saturated fat, cholesterol, and sodium) and those you want to consume in greater amounts such as dietary fiber and calcium.

Choose a percent DV of fat, saturated fat, and cholesterol less than 5 percent or as close to 5 percent as possible.

For dietary fiber, vitamins, and calcium, choose items with 20 percent or more of percent DV.

A few nutrients, like trans fat and sugar, do not have a percent DV. These are discussed below.

4. Limit intake of these items

Limit your intake of the items listed at the top of the label: total fat, saturated fat, trans fat, cholesterol, and sodium. Eating too much of these items may increase your risk of heart disease, some cancers, and high blood pressure. Check the percent DV of these items, and choose the ones with lower numbers.

- Choose low percent DV for total fat, saturated fat, and cholesterol.
- Choose a product with a low trans fat content—the smaller the better. There is no percent DV for this item, because it is not recommended even in a small amount. (Trans fat should be limited to less than 2 g a day.) Note that the trans fat level of less than 0.5 g per serving can be listed as 0 g.
- The daily allowance of sodium is 2,400 mg, or 6 g of salt. The dietary guidelines of 2010 recommend 1,500 mg per day. Uniodized salt is 40 percent sodium; therefore, the amount of sodium multiplied by 2.5 gives the amount of salt.

5. Increase intake of dietary fiber

Eating a diet high in dietary fiber promotes healthy bowel function and may reduce the risk of heart disease. The recommended daily amount of dietary fiber for adults is 25 g or more. Check the percent DV of dietary fiber when shopping.

6. Limit intake of sugar

Total carbohydrate in the nutrition facts is not important, but the amount of sugar is when buying sweet food. Too much sugar intake has been associated with becoming overweight or obese and developing diabetes. The US government has not provided the daily limit, and thus no percent DV is available.

How much sugar is too much? The Food Standards Agency (FSA) and the WHO say that no more than 10 percent of total calories should come from processed sugar:

- For a ten-year-old child and women (who need 2,000 Calories a day), the daily allowance of sugar is 200 Calories (50 g).
- For adolescent boys and young men (who need 3,000 Calories a day), the daily allowance of sugar is 300 Calories (75 g).

Get Enough of These

Get enough vitamin A, vitamin C, calcium, and iron in your diet. Choose foods with a higher percent DV of these nutrients.

Footnote

You do not need to check the footnote. This statement doesn't change from product to product. Although most of the recommendations are based on a 2,000-Calorie diet, the footnote lists daily recommended standards for both 2,000-Calorie and 2,500-Calorie diets.

Some food labels list the number of calories per gram of fat (9 Calories), carbohydrate (4 Calories) and protein (4 Calories), which are the same for every food label.

Ingredients

Some food labels show ingredients. As a rule of thumb, the fewer ingredients a product has, the healthier it is. Ingredients are listed in descending order from the greatest amount to the least. This means that food with sugar as the first or second ingredient is high in sugar and low in nutrients.

Nutrient Content Claims

The FDA provides guidelines about the claims and descriptions manufacturers may use in food labeling to promote the health benefits of their products (table 10.8). For example, to be able to claim that a product is fat-free, it should contain less than 0.5 gm of fat per serving. To claim to be a high-fiber food, it must have 5 g or more fiber per serving. The following table summarizes the requirements for frequently claimed benefits.

Table 10.8 Claims requirements for nutrition facts

Claims	Requirements that must be met before using the claim in food labeling
Fat Free	Less than 0.5 g of fat per serving, with no added fat or oil
Low Fat	3 g or less of fat per serving
Less Fat	25% or less fat than the comparison food
Saturated Fat Free	Less than 0.5 g of saturated fat and 0.5 g of tans-fatty acids per serving
Cholesterol Free	Less than 2 mg cholesterol per serving, and 2 g or less saturated fat per serving
Low Cholesterol	20 mg or less cholesterol per serving and 2 g or less saturated fat per serving
Reduced Calorie	At least 25% fewer calories per serving than the comparison food
Low Calorie	40 calories or less per serving
Lean	Less than 10 g of fat, 4.5 g of saturated fat, and 95 mg of cholesterol per (100 g) serving of meat, poultry, or seafood
Extra Lean	Less than 5 g of fat, 2 g of saturated fat, and 95 mg of cholesterol per (100 g) serving of meat, poultry, or seafood
Light (calorie)	50% or less of the fat than in the comparison food (Example: Light cheese means 50% less than regular cheese)
High Fiber	5 g or more fiber per serving
Sugar Free	Less than 0.5 g of sugar per serving
Sodium Free or Salt Free	Less than 5 mg of sodium per serving
Low Sodium	140 mg or less per serving
Very Low Sodium	35 mg or less per serving
Healthy	A food low in fat, saturated fat, cholesterol, and sodium, and that contains at least 10% of the daily Values for vitamin A, vitamin C, iron, calcium, protein, or fiber
"High," "Rich in," or "Excellent source"	20% or more of the daily Value for a given nutrient per serving
"Less," "Fewer," or "Reduced"	At least 25% less of a given nutrient or calories than the comparison food
"Low," "Little," "Few," or "Low Source of"	An amount that would allow frequent consumption of the food without exceeding the daily Value for the nutrient but can only make the claim as it applies to all similar food
"Good Source of," "More," or "Added"	The food provides 10% more of the daily Value for a given nutrient than the comparison food.

Source: FDA specifications for health claims and descriptive terms.

http://www.healthchecksystems.com/label.htm.

Chapter 11

Medications and Surgery

Medications and surgical procedures are available for adolescents with severe obesity and associated comorbidities but only at tertiary multidisciplinary obesity clinics. The information below is for your information only. If your child is severely obese and nothing seems to be working, consider taking your child to a multidisciplinary weight-management clinic to learn about possible treatments.

Medications

Many medications used to treat obesity in adults were withdrawn from the market (or their use restricted) in the past two decades because of undesirable side effects. These include fenfluramine, dexfenfluramine, ephedra, and phenylpropanolamine. These experiences underscore the need to use weight-loss medications conservatively for all obese patients and pediatric patients in particular. Aside from any potential side effects, drugs alone are not effective for weight loss, and their effects usually plateau after about six months. Weight regain is common if the drug is withdrawn. Despite these limitations, pharmacologic agents may be helpful in the treatment of obesity for carefully selected patients as part of a multimodal therapy that includes diet, exercise, and behavior modification.

Few guidelines are available regarding the use of weight-loss medications in the pediatric population. However, when clear health risks are present and lifestyle changes alone have not been effective, medications may be used as adjunctive therapy under the close supervision of experienced healthcare professionals. Children and adolescents with a BMI in the 99th percentile and higher and adults with severe obesity may be candidates for drug therapy. Presently, the FDA has approved only sibutramine and orlistat for limited use among pediatric patients. Findings of some researchers suggest that metformin, the drug approved for the treatment of insulin resistance, may improve weight control (Park et al. 2009, 1743–1745).

Meridia (Sibutramine)

Sibutramine works by boosting levels of certain chemical messengers in the nervous system by inhibiting reuptake of serotonin and norepinephrine as well as dopamine. The drug may suppress premeal hunger sensations and possibly increase RMR. It is licensed in the United States for use by persons sixteen years and older for up to two years. When used in combination with lifestyle changes (a diet and exercise program), more weight loss occurred in patients who were also taking sibutramine, but the effect plateaued after six months.

The undesirable side effects of sibutramine are increased heart rate and high blood pressure. These were observed in about 40 percent of the patients. Therefore, this drug should not be used in obese patients with associated hypertension.

Xenical (Orlistat)

Fat must be broken down to free fatty acid and glycerol by lipase before it can be absorbed into the body. Orlistat inhibits the action of lipase. In the absence of the action of lipase, fat passes through the stomach and intestine and is excreted in the feces. Through this mechanism, orlistat reduces fatty acid absorption by about 30 percent (16 g per day) in persons consuming a 30 percent fat diet. The FDA approved orlistat for patients older than twelve years of age. In 2006, the FDA recommended that orlistat be approved for over-the-counter use.

The common side effects include abdominal cramping, flatus, oily bowel movements, and oily spotting on underwear, occurring in 9 percent up to 50 percent of the patients. When a diet with more than 30 percent fat is taken, the side effects are more likely to occur. Orlistat significantly improved weight management with no major safety issues other than the adverse gastrointestinal events (Chanoine and Richard 2011, 95–101). Because it can interfere with the absorption of fat-soluble vitamins, patients taking the drug must take a daily supplement.

Metformin

In adults, metformin has been shown to reduce weight. It reduces hyperinsulinemia and hyperglycemia in obese patients with and without type 2 diabetes. There is early evidence that metformin may reduce the risk of cancer associated with obesity in adults with type 2 diabetes.

A recent meta-analysis of five publications showed that the use of metformin in obese children and adolescents had better results (reduction of BMI by 1.42) compared to a placebo control group. A small reduction in total cholesterol level was also noted. In addition, metformin was well tolerated in the adolescents. These studies suggest that metformin, in combination with a low-calorie diet, may provide modest weight loss and reduction in levels of blood sugar and insulin in adolescents who are obese and have risk factors for type 2 diabetes. However, larger studies of longer duration are needed to establish the role of metformin as a therapy for obesity and cardiometabolic risk in young people.

Bariatric Surgery

Severe obesity has proved difficult to treat through diet and lifestyle changes, even with the addition of weight-loss medications. The success of bariatric surgery to treat severe obesity with other associated conditions in adults has generated interest in using it for adolescents. At this time, information on the safety, efficacy, and long-term outcomes of bariatric surgery for adolescents is limited.

Laparoscopic Adjustable Gastric Band

The laparoscopic adjustable gastric band (LAGB) is also known as a "Lap-Band." In an LAGB procedure, the upper part of the stomach is made a small pouch by the placement of a gastric band (see fig. 11.1, left). The procedure is usually performed by laparoscopic approach. Small holes are made in the abdominal wall, and instruments are introduced through the holes rather than making a large incision in the abdominal wall. The pouch (stoma) at the top of the stomach holds approximately 110–220 g (4–7 oz.) of food. This pouch fills with food quickly and sends a message to the brain that the stomach is full, resulting in consumption of smaller portions and eventual weight loss. The gastric band is a silicone device that is inflated via a small access port placed under the skin. Saline solution is introduced into the band via the port. It decreases the size of the passage between the upper and lower parts of the stomach, further restricting the movement of food.

This procedure has not been approved by the FDA for patients younger than eighteen in the United States. It is the least invasive bariatric surgical procedure. It has the added advantages of being reversible, and the potential for adverse nutritional problems and other complications is lower than that of Roux-en-Y gastric bypass surgery. It has gained popularity in Europe and Australia. In more than 50 percent of cases, significant weight loss results in two years with minimal morbidity and almost no mortality. A recent prospective double-controlled study conducted in Australia showed that LAGB in severely obese adolescents, fourteen to eighteen years old, was better than supervised lifestyle intervention. The former approach resulted in a greater percentage of weight loss and abolishment of metabolic syndrome (Fielding and Duncombe 2005, 399–405).

Roux-en-Y Gastric Bypass

Roux-en-Y gastric bypass surgery (RYGB) is the most common bariatric surgery performed in adults and adolescents (see fig. 11.1, right). It is the only form of bariatric surgery currently approved by the FDA for use in adolescents. In this procedure, the stomach is divided into a small upper pouch and a larger lower "remnant" pouch, and both pouches are rearranged to connect to the small intestine. The middle portion of the small intestine (jenunum) is divided and the lower limb is connected to the upper pouch. The excluded lower part of the stomach and the upper part of the divided small intestine are connected to the lower jejunum at a variable distance from the pouch (fig. 11.1, right). The surgery restricts the patient's ability to overeat. Because secretions from the stomach, liver, and pancreas bypass a segment of the small bowel, food digestion is less efficient, and absorption of some nutrients is less efficient. Surgeons have developed several different ways of doing the surgery, and most centers perform it using a laparoscopic approach. In most patients, RYGB affects glycemic control (and reverses diabetes) even before weight loss occurs, whereas the effects of LAGB are dependent on weight loss.

Although many consider it the best surgical treatment for severe obesity and feel it could promote lasting weight loss for adolescent patients, there are significant complications and rare mortality rates. Complications include deficiencies of vitamins A, B1, B12, iron, and folate and inadequate absorption of calcium (resulting in hyperparathyroidism). Complications at the time of surgery may include infection, hemorrhage, and pulmonary embolism. Later on, obstruction of the small bowel, hernia at the incision site, and weight regain (in up to 15 percent of cases) may occur.

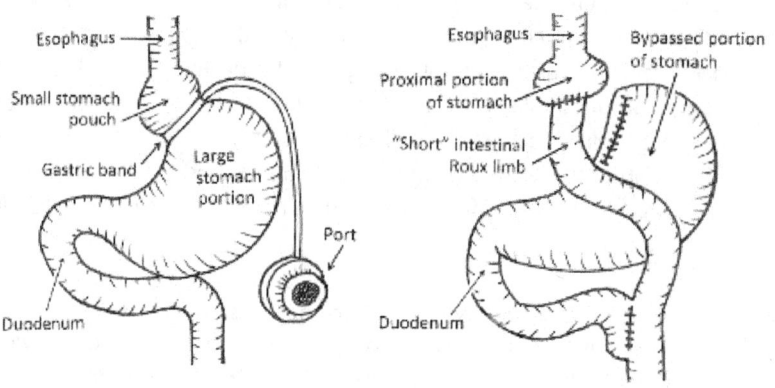

Figure 11.1. Bariatric surgical procedures. Left: Laparoscopic adjustable gastric band (LAGB). Right: Roux-en-Y gastric bypass (RYGB).

Who Is a Candidate for Bariatric Surgery?

According to the latest recommendations, the following are the selection criteria for weight-loss surgery procedures in adolescents with severe obesity (Pratt et al. 2009, 901–910).

1. Severity of obesity and comorbidities

   - BMI ≥ 35 and specific obesity-related comorbidities such as type 2 diabetes, severe steatohepatitis, pseudotumor cerebri, or moderate to severe obstructive sleep apnea
   - Extreme obesity with BMI ≥ 40 and other obesity-associated comorbidities such as mild obstructive sleep apnea, hypertension, insulin resistance, glucose intolerance, dyslipidemia, or impaired quality of life or activities of daily living

2. Failed ≥ six months of organized attempts at weight management as determined by the primary care provider

3. Attained or nearly attained physiologic maturity (generally thirteen years of age for girls and ≥ fifteen years of age for boys). For Roux-en-Y gastric bypass, near complete sexual maturation and bone age showing at least 95 percent of estimated growth are also required

4. Evidence for mature decision making with appropriate understanding of potential risks and benefits of surgery

5. Demonstrated commitment to comprehensive medical and psychological evaluation before and after surgery

6. Evidence that the family and patient have the ability and motivation to comply with the recommended treatment pre- and postoperatively

7. If a psychiatric condition (e.g., depression, anxiety, or binge-eating disorder) is present, it is under treatment

8. Agreed to avoid pregnancy for at least one year postoperatively

9. Provided informed assent to surgical treatment

In addition, the center should have an experienced bariatric surgeon and a team of specialists capable of long-term follow-up care for the metabolic and psychosocial needs of the patient and family.

Conclusion

A significant portion of adolescents with severe obesity do not succeed in medical management and many of them have significant medical complications. Adult patients with severe obesity with medical complications who underwent bariatric surgery have shown a decrease in mortality from heart disease, diabetes, and cancer. This has led physicians to, at times, recommend consideration for bariatric surgery.

LAGB appears preferable to RYGB because of its reversibility and a lower rate of complications. RYGB has higher rate of surgical complications, often more severe, and the procedure cannot be easily reversed.

For adolescents, surgery appears to result in sustained and clinically significant reduction in BMI for most patients, resolve some medical conditions including diabetes and hypertension, and reduce risk factors for diabetes and heart disease with improvement in blood sugar, cholesterol, and triglyceride levels.

Surgery should be performed only by experienced surgeons associated with a multidisciplinary pediatric obesity center. It is reserved only for those adolescents with severe obesity and significant comorbidities only after unsuccessful nonsurgical interventions. They must meet the stringent selection criteria outlined above. It should be understood that surgery does not cure obesity; even after the surgery, these adolescents will need to continue with healthy lifestyle behaviors. Some of them may need prolonged nutritional and psychological support after surgery.

Appendix

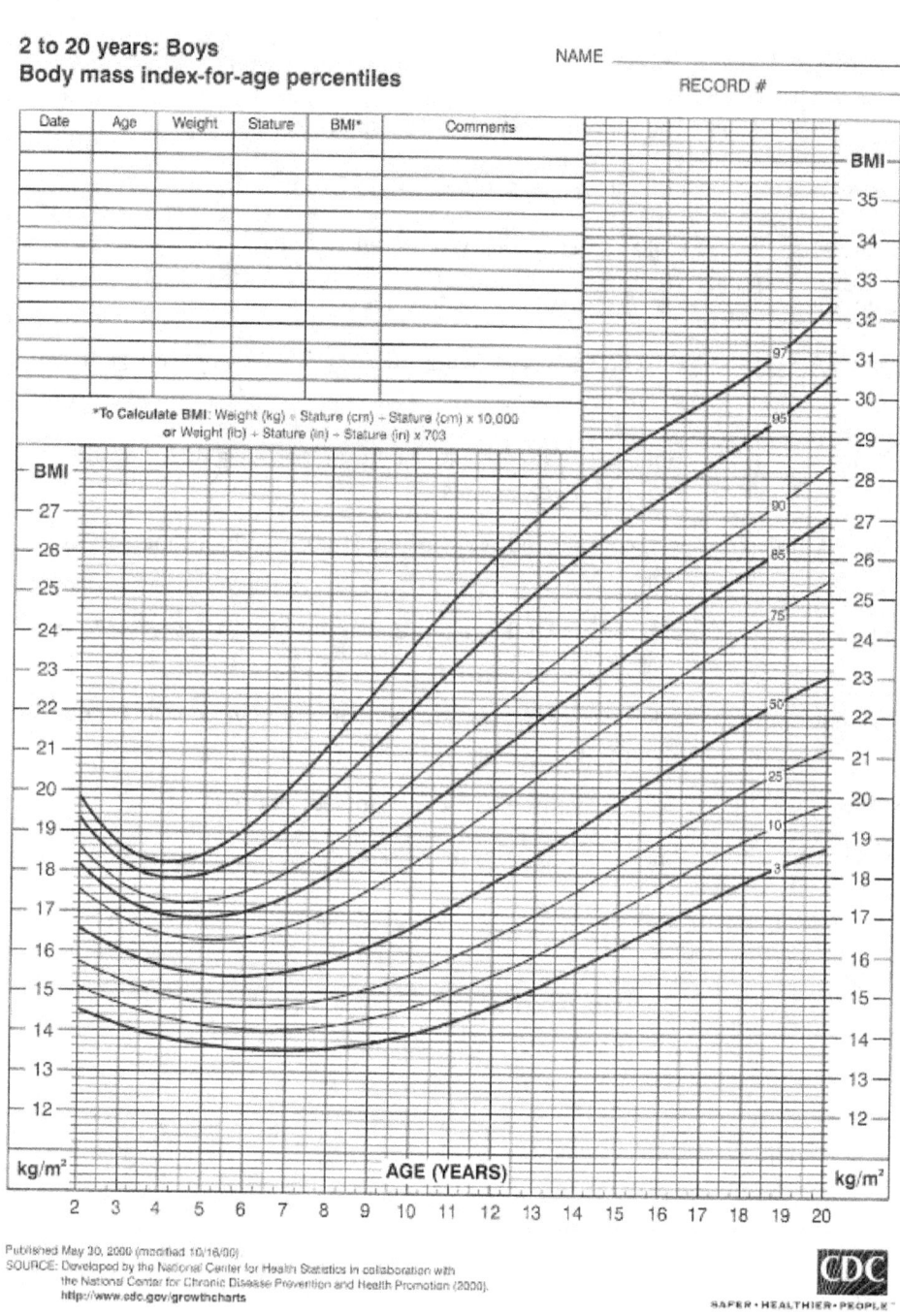

Figure A.1. BMI for Age Percentiles Two to Twenty Years: Boys

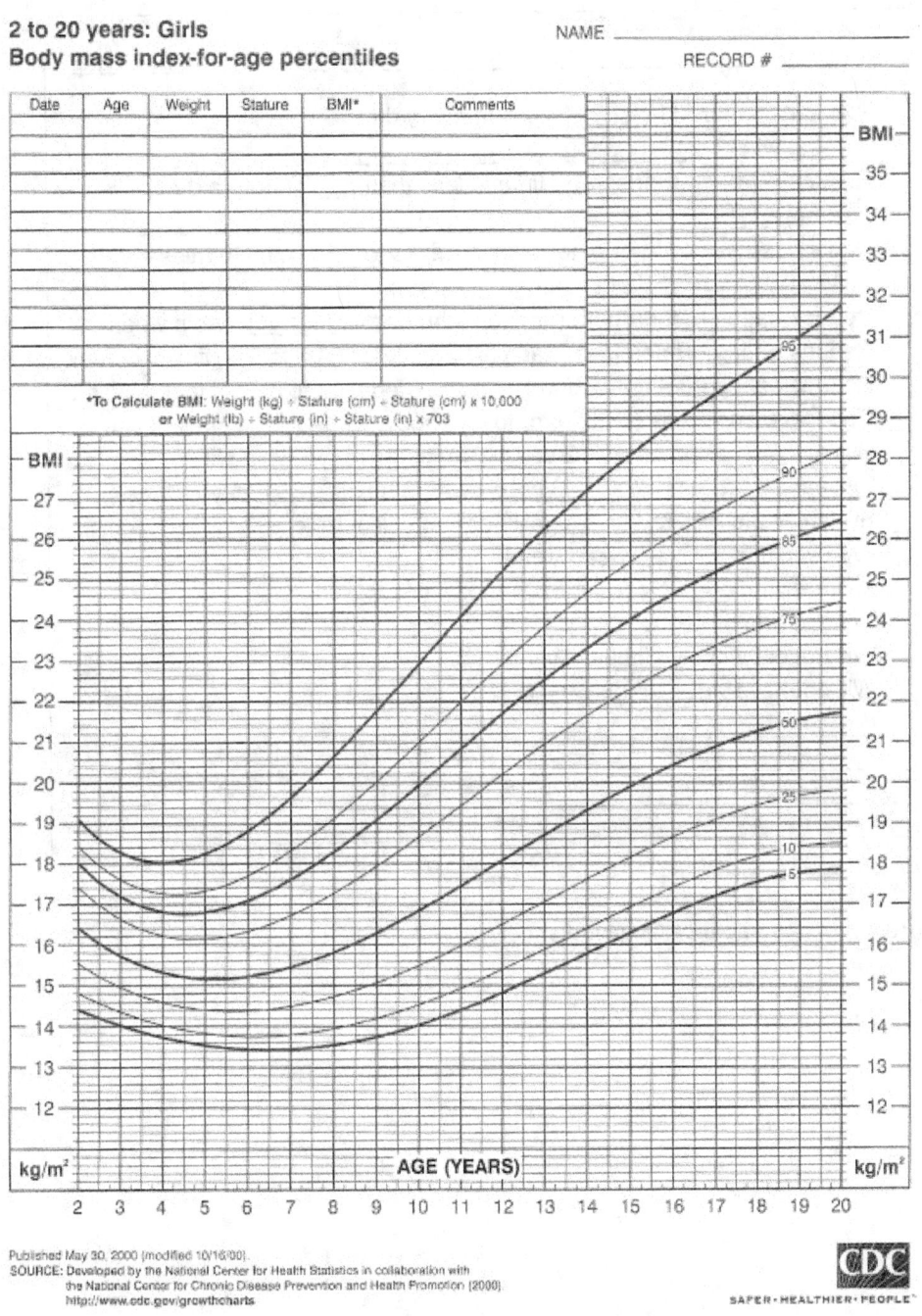

Figure A.2. BMI for Age Percentiles Two to Twenty Years: Girls

Name: _____Date: _____

____ Play outside for at least _____ min every day
Doing what? _____

____ Reduce TV and other screen time to less than _____ hours a day
(Note) _____

____ Reduce regular soda or other sugary drinks to _____ cans/bottles a day
Will drink _____ diet soda or _____ water

____ Reduce eating hamburgers (or cheeseburgers) to _____times a week

____ Reduce eating French fries (hash browns, tater tots) to _____times a week

____ Reduce eating fried foods (fried chicken, fried fish) to _____ times a week

____ Reduce eating chips (__oz bag) to __ bags a week (or ___ oz a week)

____ Will eat ___ 1 cup or ___ 2 cups of fruits _____ days a week

____ Will eat ___ 2 cups or ___ 3 cups of vegetables _____ days a week

____ Switch whole milk to ____% milk or _____ skim milk

____ Will switch to whole-wheat bread

____ Will eat whole-grain cereals for breakfast

____ Will not skip breakfast

____ Will not eat while watching TV

____ Will not have after-dinner snacks

____ _____
____ _____
____ _____
____ _____

Figure A.3. Child's goal-setting worksheet.

Date: _____

Grocery Shopping Reminders

___ Check food labels before buying foods

___ Buy more fruit and vegetables

     (Note) _____

___ Limit buying sodas

     _____ No sodas at all _____ Buy limited number _____ Buy diet sodas only

___ Limit purchase of chips

     _____ No chips ___ Limit number to _____ _____ Buy baked chips only

___ Limit high-sugar/high-fat snacks (Ice cream, cakes, cookies, etc)

     Do not buy:_____ Reduce: _____

___ Buy low-sugar varieties of: ___ ice cream, ___ cakes, ___ cookies, or _____

___ Buy lean meats and more poultry and fish

     ___ Lean meats ___ More poultry ___ More fish

___ Buy more reduced-fat dairy products

     ___ Milk, only ___%, _____ Cheese

___ Limit purchase (and cooking) of potatoes

___ _____

___ _____

Food Preparation

___ Make more meal main courses with vegetables

     (Note) _____

___ Make fruits and vegetables available as snacks

___ Do not deep fry or pan fry foods

___ Reduce serving traditional high-calorie desserts

Home and Family

___ Remove TV set from child's bedroom

___ Make house TV rule (Describe)_____

___ Limit eating restaurant foods (including take out to _____ time(s) a week

___ Have family dinners _____ time(s) a week

___ Have family outings _____ time(s) a month

___ _____

Figure A.4. Parents' goal-setting worksheet.

SUN	MON	TUE	WED	THU	FRI	SAT
1 2 3 4 5 6 CP	1 2 3 4 5 6 CP	1 2 3 4 5 6 CP	1 2 3 4 5 6 CP	1 2 3 4 5 6 CP	1 2 3 4 5 6 CP	1 2 3 4 5 6 CP
1 2 3 4 5 6 CP	1 2 3 4 5 6 CP	1 2 3 4 5 6 CP	1 2 3 4 5 6 CP	1 2 3 4 5 6 CP	1 2 3 4 5 6 CP	1 2 3 4 5 6 CP
1 2 3 4 5 6 CP	1 2 3 4 5 6 CP	1 2 3 4 5 6 CP	1 2 3 4 5 6 CP	1 2 3 4 5 6 CP	1 2 3 4 5 6 CP	1 2 3 4 5 6 CP
1 2 3 4 5 6 CP	1 2 3 4 5 6 CP	1 2 3 4 5 6 CP	1 2 3 4 5 6 CP	1 2 3 4 5 6 CP	1 2 3 4 5 6 CP	1 2 3 4 5 6 CP
1 2 3 4 5 6 CP	1 2 3 4 5 6 CP	1 2 3 4 5 6 CP	1 2 3 4 5 6 CP	1 2 3 4 5 6 CP	1 2 3 4 5 6 CP	1 2 3 4 5 6 CP

Use a circle for fully accomplished goal and a triangle for partially accomplished goal.

CP = Child-Parent Interaction

Goal Code

1 = _____

2 = _____

3 = _____

4 = _____

5 = _____

6 = _____

Figure A.5. Goal calendar and self-monitoring for weight management for six or fewer goals.

SUN	MON	TUE	WED	THU	FRI	SAT
1 2 3 4 5 6 7 8 9 10 11 12 CP	1 2 3 4 5 6 7 8 9 10 11 12 CP	1 2 3 4 5 6 7 8 9 10 11 12 CP	1 2 3 4 5 6 7 8 9 10 11 12 CP	1 2 3 4 5 6 7 8 9 10 11 12 CP	1 2 3 4 5 6 7 8 9 10 11 12 CP	1 2 3 4 5 6 7 8 9 10 11 12 CP
1 2 3 4 5 6 7 8 9 10 11 12 CP	1 2 3 4 5 6 7 8 9 10 11 12 CP	1 2 3 4 5 6 7 8 9 10 11 12 CP	1 2 3 4 5 6 7 8 9 10 11 12 CP	1 2 3 4 5 6 7 8 9 10 11 12 CP	1 2 3 4 5 6 7 8 9 10 11 12 CP	1 2 3 4 5 6 7 8 9 10 11 12 CP
1 2 3 4 5 6 7 8 9 10 11 12 CP	1 2 3 4 5 6 7 8 9 10 11 12 CP	1 2 3 4 5 6 7 8 9 10 11 12 CP	1 2 3 4 5 6 7 8 9 10 11 12 CP	1 2 3 4 5 6 7 8 9 10 11 12 CP	1 2 3 4 5 6 7 8 9 10 11 12 CP	1 2 3 4 5 6 7 8 9 10 11 12 CP
1 2 3 4 5 6 7 8 9 10 11 12 CP	1 2 3 4 5 6 7 8 9 10 11 12 CP	1 2 3 4 5 6 7 8 9 10 11 12 CP	1 2 3 4 5 6 7 8 9 10 11 12 CP	1 2 3 4 5 6 7 8 9 10 11 12 CP	1 2 3 4 5 6 7 8 9 10 11 12 CP	1 2 3 4 5 6 7 8 9 10 11 12 CP
1 2 3 4 5 6 7 8 9 10 11 12 CP	1 2 3 4 5 6 7 8 9 10 11 12 CP	1 2 3 4 5 6 7 8 9 10 11 12 CP	1 2 3 4 5 6 7 8 9 10 11 12 CP	1 2 3 4 5 6 7 8 9 10 11 12 CP	1 2 3 4 5 6 7 8 9 10 11 12 CP	1 2 3 4 5 6 7 8 9 10 11 12 CP

Use a circle for fully accomplished goal and a triangle for partially accomplished goal.

CP = Child-Parent Interaction

Goal Code

1 = _____   7 = _____
2 = _____   8 = _____
3 = _____   9 = _____
4 = _____   10 = _____
5 = _____   11 = _____
6 = _____   12 = _____

Figure A.6. Goal calendar and self-monitoring for weight management for up to twelve goals.

Table A.1(a) Body mass index (for BMI 19 to 35)

BMI Height (in.)	19	20	21	22	23	24	25	26	27	28	29	30	31	32	33	34	35
									Body Weight (lb.)								
58	91	96	100	105	110	115	119	124	129	134	138	143	148	153	158	162	167
59	94	99	104	109	114	119	124	128	133	138	143	148	153	158	163	168	173
60	97	102	107	112	118	123	128	133	138	143	148	153	158	163	168	174	179
61	100	106	111	116	122	127	132	137	143	148	153	158	164	169	174	180	185
62	104	109	115	120	126	131	136	142	147	153	158	164	169	175	180	186	191
63	107	113	118	124	130	135	141	146	152	158	163	169	175	180	186	191	197
64	110	116	122	128	134	140	145	151	157	163	169	174	180	186	192	197	204
65	114	120	126	132	138	144	150	156	162	168	174	180	186	192	198	204	210
66	118	124	130	136	142	148	155	161	167	173	179	186	192	198	204	210	216
67	121	127	134	140	146	153	159	166	172	178	185	191	198	204	211	217	223
68	125	131	138	144	151	158	164	171	177	184	190	197	203	210	216	223	230
69	128	135	142	149	155	162	169	176	182	189	196	203	209	216	223	230	236
70	132	139	146	153	160	167	174	181	188	195	202	209	216	222	229	236	243
71	136	143	150	157	165	172	179	186	193	200	208	215	222	229	236	243	250
72	140	147	154	162	169	177	184	191	199	206	213	221	228	235	242	250	258
73	144	151	159	166	174	182	189	197	204	212	219	227	235	242	250	257	265
74	148	155	163	171	179	186	194	202	210	218	225	233	241	249	256	264	272
75	152	160	168	176	184	192	200	208	216	224	232	240	248	256	264	272	279
76	156	164	172	180	189	197	205	213	221	230	238	246	254	263	271	279	287

To use the table, find the appropriate height in the left-hand column labeled Height. Move across to a given weight. The number at the top of the column is the BMI at that height and weight. Pounds have been rounded off. [From National Heart, Lung and Blood Institute, US Department of Health and Human Services http://www.nhlbi.nih.gov/health/educational/lose_wt/BMI/bmi_tbl.htm]

Table A.1(b) Body mass index (for BMI greater than 35)

Body Weight (lb.)

Height (in.) / BMI	36	37	38	39	40	41	42	43	44	45	46	47	48	49	50	51	52	53	54
58	172	177	181	186	191	196	201	205	210	215	220	224	229	234	239	244	248	253	258
59	178	183	188	193	198	203	208	212	217	222	227	232	237	242	247	252	257	262	267
60	184	189	194	199	204	209	215	220	225	230	235	240	245	250	255	261	266	271	276
61	190	195	201	206	211	217	222	227	232	238	243	248	254	259	264	269	275	280	285
62	196	202	207	213	218	224	229	235	240	246	251	256	262	267	273	278	284	289	295
63	203	208	214	220	225	231	237	242	248	254	259	265	270	276	282	287	293	299	304
64	209	215	221	227	232	238	244	250	256	262	267	273	279	285	291	296	302	308	314
65	216	222	228	234	240	246	252	258	264	270	276	282	288	294	300	306	312	318	324
66	223	229	235	241	247	253	260	266	272	278	284	291	297	303	309	315	322	328	334
67	230	236	242	249	255	261	268	274	280	287	293	299	306	312	319	325	331	338	344
68	236	243	249	256	262	269	276	282	289	295	302	308	315	322	328	335	341	348	354
69	243	250	257	263	270	277	284	291	297	304	311	318	324	331	338	345	351	358	365
70	250	257	264	271	278	285	292	299	306	313	320	327	334	341	348	355	362	369	376
71	257	265	272	279	286	293	301	308	315	322	329	338	343	351	358	365	372	379	386
72	265	272	279	287	294	302	309	316	324	331	338	346	353	361	368	375	383	390	397
73	272	280	288	295	302	310	318	325	333	340	348	355	363	371	378	386	393	401	408
74	280	287	295	303	311	319	326	334	342	350	358	365	373	381	389	396	404	412	420
75	287	295	303	311	319	327	335	343	351	359	367	375	383	391	399	407	415	423	431
76	295	304	312	320	328	336	344	353	361	369	377	385	394	402	410	418	426	435	443

To use the table, find the appropriate height in the left-hand column labeled Height. Move across to a given weight. The number at the top of the column is the BMI at that height and weight. Pounds have been rounded off.
[From National Heart, Lung and Blood Institute, US Department of Health and Human Services http://www.nhlbi.nih.gov/health/educational/lose_wt/BMI/bmi_tbl.htm]

Table A.2 Selected percentile values of body mass index (BMI) for boys and girls 4 to 20 years of age*

	Boys					Girls			
Age (yr.)	50th percentile	85th percentile	95th percentile	99th percentile†	Age (yr.)	50th percentile	85th percentile	95th percentile	99th percentile†
4	15.6	16.9	17.9		4	15.3	16.8	18.0	
5	15.4	16.8	17.9	20.6	5	15.2	16.8	18.3	21.5
6	15.4	17.0	18.4	21.6	6	15.3	17.1	18.8	23.0
7	15.5	17.4	19.2	23.6	7	15.5	17.6	19.7	24.6
8	15.8	17.9	20.0	25.6	8	15.8	18.3	20.7	26.4
9	16.2	18.6	21.1	27.6	9	16.3	19.1	21.8	28.2
10	16.6	19.3	22.2	29.3	10	16.8	19.9	22.9	29.9
11	17.2	20.2	23.2	30.7	11	17.4	20.8	24.1	31.5
12	17.8	21.0	24.2	31.8	12	18.1	21.7	25.2	33.1
13	18.4	21.8	25.2	32.6	13	18.7	22.5	26.3	34.6
14	19.1	22.6	26.0	33.2	14	19.3	23.3	27.3	36.0
15	19.8	23.4	26.8	33.6	15	19.9	24.0	28.1	37.5
16	20.5	24.2	27.5	33.9	16	20.4	24.7	28.8	39.1
17	21.2	24.9	28.2	34.4	17	20.9	25.2	29.6	40.8
18	21.8	25.6	28.9		18	21.3	25.7	30.3	
19	22.5	26.3	29.7		19	21.5	26.1	31.0	
20	23.0	27.0	30.5		20	21.7	26.5	31.8	

*Tabularized from the normative percentile curves published by the National Center for Disease Prevention and Health Promotion (2000).

† The 99th percentile values are from the expert committee summary report 2007.

Modified from B. A. Spear, et al., "Recommendations for treatment of child and adolescent overweight and obesity." *Pediatrics* 120, suppl. 4 (2007): S254–S288.

Table A.3 Genetic syndromes associated with obesity

Syndrome	Clinical symptoms and signs
Prader-Willi syndrome	• Infantile hypotonia • Poor feeding initially followed by striking hyper-phagia and weight gain • Developmental delay • Short stature • Small hands and feet • Behavioral and psychosocial problems
Bardet-Biedl syndrome	• Polydactyly • Mental retardation • Short stature • Retinitis pigmentosa • Renal disease • Hypogonadism
Alström syndrome	• Nerve deafness • Diabetes • Pigmentary retinal degeneration • Cataracts
Albright hereditary osteodystrophy	• Short stature • May have pseudohypoparathyroidism • Ectopic calcifications • Hypocalcemia
Hereditary Cushing syndrome	• Carney complex: an autosomal dominant syndrome of multiple neoplasia (cardiac, endocrine, cutaenous and neural tumors), spotty skin pigmented lesions of skin and mucosa, multiple endocrine neoplasia (pituitary adenomas or testicular tumors) • Testicular hypoplasia • Ovarian cysts
Isolated growth hormone deficiency	• Short stature • Central obesity
X-linked syndromic mental retardation	• X-linked mental retardation • High prevalence of obesity from mutations in the MECP2 gene

Modified from S. G. Hassink, *"Pediatric Obesity. Prevention, Intervention, and Treatment Strategies for Primary Care."* (Elk Grove Viillage, IL. American Academy of Pediatrics, 2007)

NOTE: Most genetic conditions associated with obesity have in common mental retardation and short stature.

Box A.1 One hundred ways to praise a child

• Hey, I love you! • Way to go! • You're special! • Outstanding! • Excellent! • You are fun! • You're a real trooper! • You're on target! • Outstanding performance! • Great!	• You are the clever one! • You are just delightful! • That's incredible! • Remarkable job! • You're Beautiful! • You're a winner! • You make me happy! • Dynamite! • Hip, Hip, Hooray! • You're important!	• Super work! • You mean a lot to me! • You're a good friend! • You deserve a big hug! • You are an absolute gem! • You're incredible! • I like you! • Now you're flying! • I respect you! • You're sensational!
• Looking good! • You brighten my day! • Good! • Well done! • Remarkable! • Super! • I knew you could do it! • Nice work! • What an imagination! • I'm proud of you!	• Magnificent! • Beautiful! • Super job! • You're the best! • You're on your way! • How nice! • You're Spectacular! • You are a Darling! • Beautiful work! • Good for you!	• Phenomenal! • Hooray for you! • You care! • Creative job! • You belong! • You made my day! • You are nice to be with! • You mean the world to me! • You're important! • You've got a friend!
• Super star! • Fantastic! • You're on top of it! • You're catching on! • Now you've got it! • How smart! • Good job! • Remarkable! • Super! • I knew you could do it!	• Nothing can stop you now! • You're fantastic! • Wow! • You're a legend! • Great Discovery! • Fantastic job! • You're a champion! • Awesome! • You're precious! • Marvelous!	• You're a joy! • You make me laugh! • You're A-OK! • You're my buddy! • I trust you! • You're perfect! • Bravo! • You're wonderful! • A big kiss! • Exceptional performance!
• Nice work! • What an imagination! • I'm proud of you! • Superstar! • Fantastic! • You're on top of it! • You're catching on! • Now you've got it! • How smart! • Good job!	• You are responsible! • Terrific! • You are exciting! • You're growing up! • You tried hard! • Neat! • You figured it out! • You're unique! • What a good listener! • You're a treasure!	• That's correct! • You've discovered the secret! **♥ PS. Remember a HUG is worth 1000 words! ♥**

With compliments from the Fatherhood Foundation, PO Box 440, Wollongong, NSW 2520, Australia. Website: www.fathersonline.org.

Notes

References are arranged by the last name of the first author for journal articles and by the name of the first organization for website information.

American Academy of Pediatrics, Committee on Public Education. 2000–2001. "Children, Adolescents, and Television." http://pediatrics.aappublications.org/content/107/2/423.full.

Baranowski, T., M. Smith, M. D. Hearn, et al. 1997. "Patterns in children's fruit and vegetable consumption by meal and day of the week." *Journal of American College of Nutrition* 16: 216–223.

Barlow, S. E., and the Expert Committee. 2007. "Expert committee recommendations regarding the prevention, assessment, and treatment of child and adolescent overweight and obesity: Summary report." *Pediatrics* 120: S164–S192.

Berkey, C. S., H. R. Rockett, M. W. Gilman, A. E. Field, et al. 2003. "Longitudinal study of skipping breakfast and weight change in adolescents." *International Journal of Obesity and Related Metabolic Disorders* 27: 1258–1266.

Bibbin-Domingo, K., G. M. Chertow, P. G. Coxson, A. Moran, et al. 2010. "Projected effect of dietary salt reduction on future cardiovascular disease." *New England Journal of Medicine* 362, no. 7: 590–599.

Bowman, S. A., S. L. Gortmaker, C. B. Ebbeling, M. A. Pereira, et al. 2004. "Effects of fast-food consumption on energy intake and diet quality among children in a national household survey." *Pediatrics* 113: 112–118.

Brand-Miller, J. C., S. H. A. Holt, D. B. Pawlak, and J. McMillan. 2002. "Glycemic index and obesity." *American Journal of Clinical Nutrition* 76, suppl.: 281S–285S.

Bravata, D. M., C. Smith-Spangler, V. Sundaram, A. L. Gienger, et al. 2007. "Using pedometers to increase physical activity and improve health: a systematic review." *Journal of American Medical Association* 298, no. 19: 296–304.

Cash, H., C. D. Rae, A. H. Steel, and A. Winkler. 2012. "Internet addiction: A brief summary of research and practice." *Current Psychiatry Reviews* 8, no. 4: 292–298.

Center for Disease Control and Prevention. December 2009. "Nutrition and the Health of Young People." http://www.cdc.gov/healthyyouth/nutrition/facts.htm.

Chanoine, J. P., and M. Richard. 2011. "Early weight loss and outcome at one year in obese adolescents treated with orlistat or placebo." *International Journal of Pediatric Obesity* 6: 95–101.

Crespo, C. J., E. Smit, R. P. Troiano, S. J. Bartless, et al. 2001. "Television watching, energy intake, and obesity in US children." *Journal of American Medical Association* 155: 360–365.

Cuo, S. S., and W. C. Chumlea. 1999. "Tracking of body mass index in children in relation to overweight in adulthood." *American Journal of Clinical Nutrition* 70, Suppl.: 145S–148S.

Dietz, W. H., L. G. Bandini, J. A. Morelli, K. F. Peers, et al. 1994. "Effects of sedentary activities on resting metabolic rate." *American Journal of Clinical Nutrition* 59, no. 9: 556–559.

Donin, A. S., C. M. Nightingale, C. G. Owen, A. R. Rudnicka, et al. 2014. "Regular breakfast consumption and type 2 diabetes risk markers in 9- to 10-year-old children in the child heart and Health Study in England (CHASE): A cross-sectional analysis." *Public Library of Science Medicine* 11, no. 9: e1001703.

Environmental Working Group. July 21, 2003. "PCB in farmed salmon." http://www.ewg.org/research/pcbs-farmed-salmon.

Epstein, L. H., A. Valoski, R. R. Wing, and J. McCurley. 1994. "Ten-year outcome of behavioral family-based treatment for childhood obesity." *Health Psychology* 13, no. 5: 373–383.

Ervin, R. B., B. K. Kit, M. D. Carroll, and C. L. Ogden. 2012. "Consumption of added sugar among U.S. children and adolescents, 2005–2008." NCHS data brief, no. 87 (Hyattsville, MD: National Center for Health Statistics).

Fielding, G. A., and J. E. Duncombe. 2005. "Laparoscopic adjustable gastric banding in severely obese adolescents." *Surgery for Obesity and Related Diseases* 1, no. 4: 399–405.

Fowler, S. P., K. William, R. G. Resendez, K. J. Hunt, et al. 2008. "Fueling the obesity epidemic? Artificially sweetened beverage use and long-term weight gain." *Obesity* 16, no. 8: 1894–1900.

Germann, J. N., D. S. Kirschenbaum, and B. H. Rich. 2007. "Child and parental self-monitoring as determinants of success in the treatment of morbid obesity in low-income minority children." *Journal of Pediatric Psychology* 32, no. 1: 111–121.

Gillman, M. W., S. L. Rifas-Shiman, A. L. Frazier, H. R. Rockett, et al. 2000. "Family dinner and diet quality among older children and adolescents." *Archives of Family Medicine 9*: 235–240.

Gini, G., and T. Pozzoli. 2009. "Association between bullying and psychosomatic problems: a meta analysis," *Pediatrics* 123: 1059–1065.

Golan, M., A. Weizman, A. Apter, and M. Fainaru. 1998. "Parents as the exclusive agents of change in the treatment of childhood obesity." *American Journal of Clinical Nutrition* 67:1130–1135.

Golan, M., A. Weizman, and M. Fainaru. 1999. "Impact of treatment for childhood obesity on parental risk for cardiovascular disease." *Preventive Medicine* 6: 519–526.

Green Philly. June 2013. "Why is farm raised fish so bad?" http://www.greenphillyblog.com/green-living/reader-question-why-is-farm-raised-so-bad/.

Hammons, A. J., and B. H. Fiese. 2011. "Is frequency of shared family meals related to the nutritional health of children and adolescents?" *Pediatrics* 127, no. 6: e1565–1574.

He, F. J., and G. A. MacGregor. 2010. "Reducing population salt intake worldwide: from evidence to implementation," *Progress in Cardiovascular Diseases* 52: 363–382.

Hellerstein, M. K. 2002. "Carbohydrate-induced hypertriglyceridemia: modifying factors and implications for cardiovascular risk." *Current Opinion in Lipidology* 13, no. 1: 33–40.

Hoyland, A., L. Dye, and C. L. Lawton. 2009. "A systematic review of the effect of breakfast on the cognitive performance of children and adolescents." *Nutrition Research Review* 22: 220–243.

Janssen, I., W. Craig, W. Boyce, and W. Pickett. 2004. "Association between overweight and obesity with bully behaviors in school-aged children." *Pediatrics* 113, no. 5: 1187–1194.

Jenkins, D. J. A., T. M. S. Wolever, R. H. Taylor, H. Barker, et al. 1981. "Glycemic index of foods: a physiological basis for carbohydrate exchange." *American Journal of Clinical Nutrition* 34: 362–366.

Kelishadi, R., M. Mansourian, and M. Heidari-Beni. 2014. "Association of fructose consumption and components of metabolic syndrome in human studies: a systematic review and meta-analysis." *Nutrition* 30, no. 5: 503–510.

Kritchevsky, S. B. 2004. "A review of scientific research and recommendations regarding eggs." *Journal of American College of Nutrition* 23, 6 suppl.: 596S–600S.

Laurson, K. R., J. C. Eisenmann, G. L. Welk, E. E. Wickel, et al. 2008. "Evaluation of youth pedometer-determined physical activity guidelines using receiver operator character= istic curves." *Preventive Medicine* 46 no. 5: 419–424.

Ludwig, D. S., J. A. Majzoub, A. Al-Zahrani, G. E. Dallal, et al. 1999. "High glycemic index foods, overeating, and obesity." *Pediatrics* 103: E261–E266.

Manco, M., G. Bottazzo, R. Devito, M. Marcellini, et al. 2008. "Nonalcoholic fatty liver disease in children: Review." *Journal of American College of Nutrition* 27, no. 6: 667–676.

Margarey, A. M., R. A. Perry, L. A. Baur, K. S. Steinbeck, et al. 2011. "A parent-led family-focused treatment program for overweight children aged 5 to 9 years: the PEACH RCT." *Pediatrics* 127: 214–222.

Mattillo, S., K. B. Filion, J. Genest, L. Josphe, et al. 2010. "The metabolic syndrome and cardiovascular risk: A systematic review and meta-analysis." *Journal of American College of Cardiology* 56: 1113–1132.

Mozaffarian, D., T. Hao, E. B. Rimm, W. C. Willett, et al. 2011. "Changes in diet and lifestyle and long-term weight gain in women and men." *New England Journal of Medicine* 364: 2392–2404.

Mozaffarian, D., M. Katan, A. Ascherio, M. Stampfer, et al. 2006. "Trans fatty acids and cardiovascular disease." *New England Journal of Medicine* 354: 1601–1613.

National Cancer Institute. July 2008. "Acrylamide in Food and Cancer Risk." http://www.cancer.gov/cancertopics/factsheet/Risk/acrylamide-in-food

National Center for Chronic Disease Prevention and Health Promotion, Research to Practice Series, No. 5. 2010. "Low-energy-dense foods and weight management: cutting calories while controlling hunger." Washington, DC. http://www.cdc.gov/nccdphp/dnpa/nutrition/pdf/r2p_energy_density.pdf.

National Crime Prevention Council. "What parents can do: Advice for parents and adults about how to deal with bullying." http://www.ncpc.org/topics/bullying/what-parents-can-do.

Neumark-Sztainer, D., P. L. Hannan, M. Story, J. Croll, et al. 2003. "Family meal patterns: Associations with sociodemographic characteristics and improved dietary intake among adolescents." *Journal of American Dietetic Association 103*: 317–322.

Ogden, C. L., M. D. Carroll, B. K. Kit, and K. M. Flegal. 2014. "Prevalence of childhood and adult obesity in the United States, 2011–2012." *Journal of American Medical Association* 311: 806–816.

Park, M. H., S. Kinra, K. J. Ward, B. White, R. M. Viner. 2009. "Metformin for obesity in children and adolescents: a systemic review." *Diabetes Care* 32: 1743–1745.

Pratt, J. S. A., C. M. Lenders, E. A. Dionne, A. G. Hoppin, et al. 2009. "Best practice update for pediatric/adolescent weight loss surgery." *Obesity* 17: 901–910.

Prochaska, J. O., C. C. DiClemente, and J. C. Norcross. 1992. "In search of how people change: Applications to addictive behavior." *American Psychologist* 47, no. 9: 1102–1114.

Reeves, G. M., T. T. Postolache, and S. Snitker. 2008. "Childhood obesity and depression: Connection between these growing problems in growing children." *International Journal of Child Health and Human Development* 1, no. 2: 103–114.

Reicks, M., S. Jonnalagadda, A. M. Albertson, and N. Joshi. 2014. "Total dietary fiber intakes in the US population are related to whole grain consumption: results from the National Health and Nutrition Examination Survey 2009 to 2010." *Nutrition Research* 34, no. 3: 226–234.

Robinson, T. N. 1999. "Reducing children's television viewing to prevent obesity: a randomized controlled trial." *Journal of American Medical Association* 282: 1561–1567.

Schulze, M. B., J. E. Manson, D. S. Ludwig, et al. 2004. "Sugar sweetened beverages, weight gain, and incidence of type 2 diabetes in young and middle-aged women." *Journal of American Medical Association* 292: 927–934.

Sen, B. 2010. "The relationship between frequency of family dinner and adolescent problem behaviors after adjusting for other family characteristics." *Journal of Adolescence* 33, no.1: 187-196.

Singh, G. K. 2006. "Metabolic syndrome in children and adolescents." *Current Treatment Options in Cardiovascular Medicine* 8, no. 5: 403–413.

Sinha, R., A. J. Cross, B. I. Graubard, M. F. Leitzmann, et al. 2009. "Meat intake and mortality: a prospective study of over half a million people." *Archives of Internal Medicine* 169, no. 6: 562–571.

Spear, B. A., S. E. Barlow, C. Ervin, D. S. Ludwig, et al. 2007. "Recommendations for treatment of child and adolescent overweight and obesity." *Pediatrics* 120, suppl.: S254–S288.

Thompson, O. M., C. Ballew, K. Resnicow, et al. 2004. "Food purchased away from home as a predictor of change in MBI z-score among girls." *International Journal of Obesity and Related Metabolic Disorders* 28: 282–289.

Troiano, R. P., R. R. Briefel, M. D. Carroll, and K. Bialososky. 2000. "Energy and fat intakes of children and adolescents in the United States: data from the National Health and Nutrition Examination Survey." *American Journal of Clinical Nutrition* 72, Suppl.: 1343S–1353S.

United States Secret Service and United States Department of Education. May 2002. "The final report and findings of the safe school initiative: Implications for the prevention of school attacks in the United States." Washington, DC. http://www.secretservice.gov/ntac/ssi_final_report.pdf.

van der Horst, K., S. Kremers, I. Ferreira, A. Singh, et al. 2006. "Perceived parenting style and practices and the consumption of sugar-sweetened beverages by adolescents." *Health Education Research* 22, no. 2: 295–304.

Vartiainen, E., C, Sarti, J. Tuomilehto, and K. Kuulasmaa. 1995. "Do changes in cardiovascular risk factors explain changes in mortality from stroke in Finland?" *British Medical Journal* 310: 901–904.

Vartanian, L. R., M. B. Schwartz, and K. D. Brownell. 2007. "Effects of soft drink consumption on nutrition and health: A systemic review and meta-analysis." *American Journal of Public Health* 97: 667–675.

Vreeman, R., and A. Carroll., (2007). "A systematic review of School-Based interventions to prevent bullying: review article." *Archives of Pediatrics and Adolescent Medicine* 161: 78–88.

WebMD News Archive. March 15, 2010. "School lunches linked to kids' obesity." http://www.webmd.com/children/news/20100315/school-lunches-linked-to-kids-obesity.

Wiecha, J. L., K. E. Peterson, D. S. Ludwig, J. Kim, et al. 2006. "When children eat what they watch: impact of television viewing on dietary intake in youth." *Archive of Pediatric and Adolescent Medicine* 160, no. 4: 436–442.

Willett, W. C. 2005. "Fish: Balancing health risks and benefits." *American Journal of Preventive Medicine* 29, no. 4: 320–321.